# The Comfort & Healing Companion

A Patient and Caregiver Toolkit
for Treatment, Recovery, and Beyond

Thomas Kealey, RN & Lindsey Kealey, MAT

THE BRAIN IT ON! Podcast

To every patient and caregiver navigating the unexpected,
may this guide help you find moments of peace and power in the storm.

The Comfort & Healing Companion: A Patient and Caregiver Toolkit for Treatment, Recovery, and Beyond

First Edition


Published by PAWsitive Choices, LLC, Bend, OR, USA



Written by Thomas Kealey, RN & Lindsey Kealey, MAT
ISBN: 978-1-956523-16-4

Medical Disclaimer: The information in this workbook is for educational purposes only and is not intended to replace professional medical advice, diagnosis, or treatment. Always seek the advice of your physician or other qualified health provider with any questions regarding a medical condition.

# Table of Contents

# Our Story

We're Thomas and Lindsey Kealey, a husband-and-wife team and the hosts of The Brain it On! Podcast. In our professional lives, Thomas is a registered nurse and Lindsey is an instructor of Human Development and Family Sciences at Oregon State University.

**In 2024, our lives were deeply impacted when Thomas' mom was diagnosed with pancreatic cancer, just three months before Thomas himself was diagnosed with a rare, high-risk leukemia that required a bone marrow transplant.**

These back-to-back challenges plunged us into a world of complex medical realities—from navigating insurance and disability leave, to managing chemotherapy and radiation side effects. But the journey also highlighted the immense importance of **nurturing emotional well-being and finding moments of normalcy and joy amidst the clinical environment.**

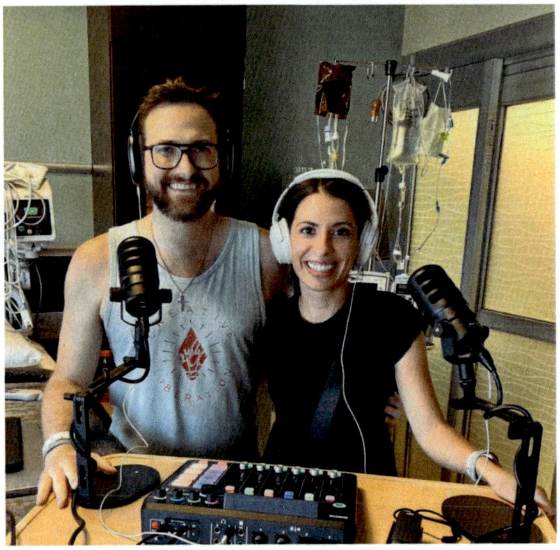

It was these personal experiences that inspired us to start The Brain it On! Podcast right from our hospital room. We wanted to share the lessons we learned and the practical strategies that made a real difference for us. This toolkit was born directly from that desire, offering resources we relied on or wished we'd known about sooner. Our hope is to empower you to **find comfort, control, and peace during your own challenging times**, transforming difficult moments into opportunities for strength.

Thanks for letting us help you on your journey!

*Thomas & Lindsey*

# Information About This Guide

Welcome to The Brain it On! Podcast's Comfort & Healing Companion. This resource is born from our personal journey and the invaluable lessons we learned navigating complex medical challenges—including Thomas' leukemia and bone marrow transplant and his mother's pancreatic cancer treatment.

We've filled these pages with the resources, comfort items, and practical strategies that made a real difference for us. Many of these items were suggested by Thomas' own oncologists and medical specialists, proving their utility in a clinical setting.

**As you explore this guide, please keep the following in mind:**

- **For Informational Purposes Only:** The information shared here reflects our personal experiences. It is not intended to be a substitute for professional medical advice, diagnosis, or treatment.

- **Consult Your Medical Team:** Always consult with your own healthcare providers before making decisions related to your care, diet, or treatment plan. They are best equipped to provide advice tailored to your specific needs.

- **Our Recommendations:** Throughout this book, you will find QR codes to curated lists with hyperlinks for our most-used comfort and wellness items. These include essentials recommended by our care team that we ordered off Amazon for delivery to the hospital. Use these lists to pack what you have, create an Amazon Wishlist, or text links to loved ones asking how to help. Choose brands that suit you best, and as always, ensure any new items align with your medical team's guidelines.

## Your Digital Resource Library

This guide is paired with an exclusive online library. We have gathered all our printable trackers, video tutorials, podcast episodes, and product links in one easy-to-access place so you can stay organized throughout your journey.

To access these resources, scan the QR code or visit:
**www.comfortandhealing.org/resources**

# DO THE NEXT RIGHT THING.

PART 1

# Navigating First Steps

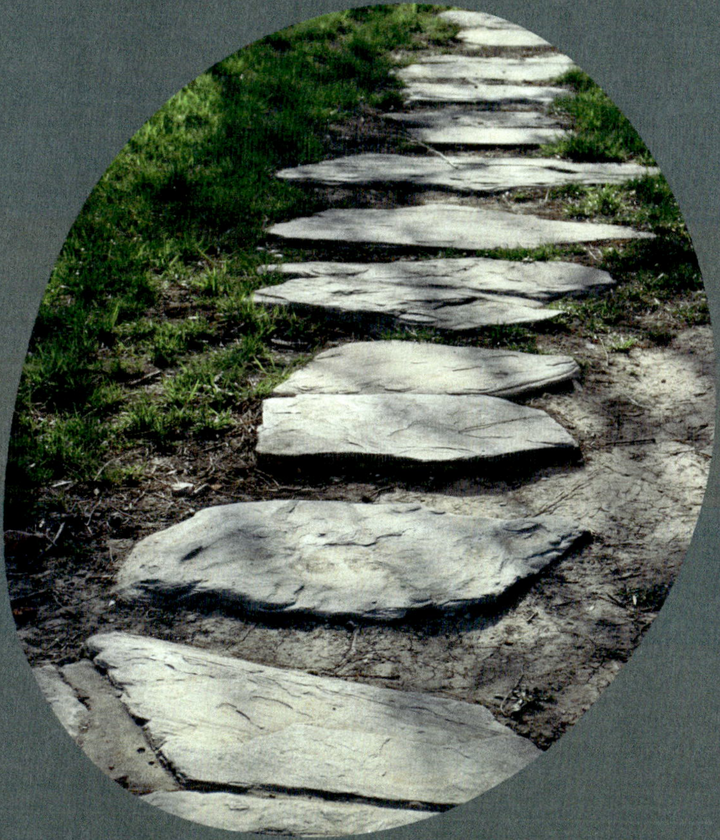

Important Information

# Starting Your Journey

A diagnosis can feel like the ground is shifting beneath your feet.

Whether you just received your diagnosis and are preparing for what's next, or you are already sitting in a hospital room, this guide is designed to meet you exactly where you are.

**Here is what we know for sure: You are stronger than you think.**

At The Brain it On! Podcast, we talk about how the brain has an incredible capacity to adapt and build **resilience**. But right now, your brain is likely on information overload. Think of this section as your "external hard drive"—a place to catch your breath, offload the logistics, and regain a sense of control so your brain can focus on healing.

**You Are Not Alone.**

There will be days when you feel overwhelmed. There will be days when your biggest "win" is taking a shower or eating your first solid food (Thomas has been there). But as you use these pages to track your progress and advocate for your needs, you are doing something powerful: **you are building resilience.**

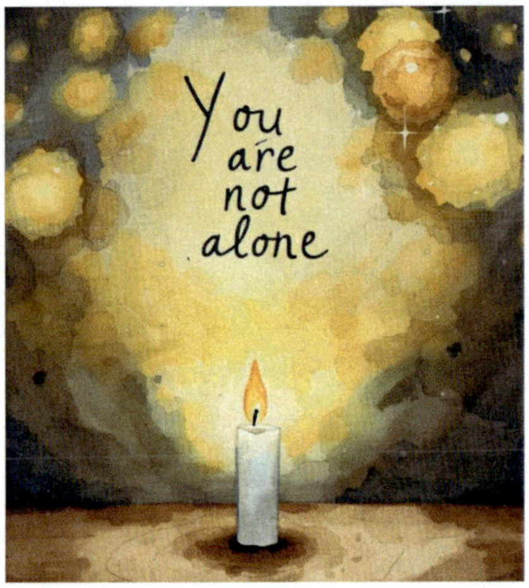


**Use these tools to ground yourself:**

- **Befriend Your Team**: Your doctors, nurses, and medical staff are your greatest allies. Use the *Who's Who: Your Hospital Village* page to understand their roles and the *Care Team Connections* pages to learn their names and build a partnership with them.
- **Learn the Language**: Don't let the jargon intimidate you. We've included pages for *Medical Terms* and *Oncology/Hematology Terms* to help you translate "doctor speak" into plain English so you can participate more confidently. Learn important employment and insurance terminology on the *Questions for Your Social Worker* page.
- **Create Your Safe Space**: Your environment matters. Use the *Hospital Packing List* to bring in "glimmers" of comfort that make a sterile room feel a little more like home.
- **Advocate for Your Needs**: You are the expert on you. Use the *Questions for Your Medical Team* page to ensure your medical concerns are heard and your questions are answered.

# Questions for Your Medical Team

Use this list as your "cheat sheet" to ensure you understand the plan. If you hear a term you don't know, check the Medical Terms glossary on the following pages. You can always ask your provider to pause, explain again, or provide printed handouts for you to read later.

**The Big Picture:**

- What is the specific name/type of my diagnosis?
- What is the stage or severity? Has it spread?
- What caused this?
- We value your expertise. For a journey this complex, do you have colleagues or other institutions you collaborate with for second opinions or clinical trials that we should be aware of?

**The Immediate Goal:**

- What is the primary goal of this first phase of treatment? (e.g., Remission, Stabilization, Symptom Management?)
- What is the 'Standard of Care'?
- What are the side effects?
- How will we know if the treatment is working? (e.g., Will we do another bone marrow biopsy, a PET scan, or just check blood counts?)

**The Timeline:**

- How soon do I need to start treatment?
- What is the estimated length of this hospital stay/treatment phase?
- How much time do I (and my caregiver) need to take off of work?

**Points of Contact**

- Who should I reach out to if I have specific medical questions?
- Who do I talk to regarding financial logistics and support?
- Who do I call if I have an emergency after-hours, on holidays, or during the weekend?

**The Milestones:**

- What specific numbers (like ANC or Platelets) do we need to hit to move to the next phase or to be discharged from the hospital?

**Morning Rounds in the Hospital:**

- What is the 'goal for the day' to get me closer to discharge? (This helps you focus on small wins, like walking a certain distance or hitting a specific lab number).
- What do my 'Big Three' labs (ANC, HGB, Platelets) look like today? (Ask if you are approaching a Transfusion Trigger).
- Are we making any changes to my meds (like IV nutrition or pain control) based on my vitals?
- Are there any tests, scans, or procedures scheduled for today that I need to be ready for?

# Questions for Your Social Worker, Case Manager, or HR Rep

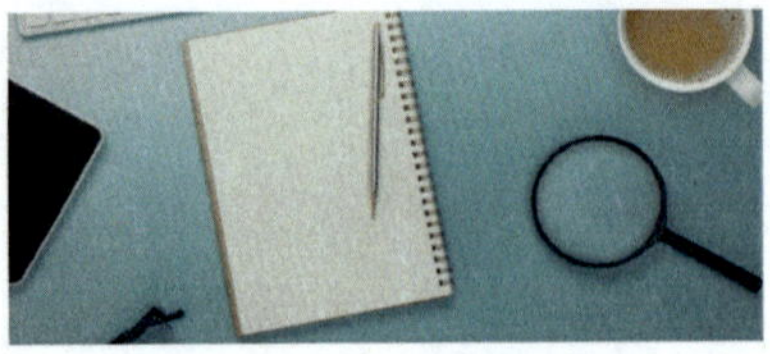

Social Workers and Case Managers are experts at connecting you with vital resources—from financial grants to counseling. Since you will receive important documents, start a binder today to keep everything organized. If they refer you to another department, always ask for a specific name and direct phone number to save time later. Use the template on the next page to keep all these critical contacts in one place.

- **Insurance & Finance:** Is there a financial coordinator who can help us understand our out-of-pocket costs and deductible? Do I qualify for Medicaid (e.g., Oregon Health Plan)? Can Medicaid work as a 'secondary' insurance to cover my deductibles?

- **Employment Protection:** Who handles the paperwork for FMLA (Family and Medical Leave Act), Short-Term Disability (STD), Long-Term Disability (LTD), and PFML (Paid Family Medical Leave)?

- **Social Security Disability Insurance (SSDI):** Do I qualify for SSDI and how do I apply? Is my condition on the Compassionate Allowances (CAL) list? If your condition is on the list, this can expedite the process.

- **COBRA:** COBRA is a federal law that lets you keep the exact same health insurance you had at your job after you leave or lose your position. Ask about specific details on COBRA enrollment deadlines, premium costs, and paperwork. Inquire about "disability COBRA" if you qualify for SSDI (this can add 11 months to your COBRA coverage).

- **Health Insurance Premium Payment (HIPP) Programs:** Who do I contact regarding a HIPP program? This is a specialized financial assistance program that can actually pay your COBRA premiums for you if it is cheaper for the state than putting you on standard Medicaid (e.g., Oregon Health Plan).

- **Housing & Travel:** Does the hospital have partnerships with local hotels or housing (like Ronald McDonald House) for long-term stays? Are there laundry facilities available on the unit for patients and families?

- **Hospital Grants:** Are there specific grants available for parking, meal vouchers, or travel assistance?

- **Mental Health:** What support services (counseling, support groups, or chaplaincy) are available for both the patient and the caregiver?

# The Master List: Insurance & Employment

Keep this page handy for every phone call. Pro tip: Take a clear photo of the front and back of every insurance and ID card. Save them in a specific 'Medical' album on your phone so you have them even if you forget your wallet.

**1. MEDICAL INSURANCE**

**Primary Insurance Company:** ____________________

- **Member ID #:** ____________________ **Group #:** ____________________
- **Plan Type (PPO/HMO/etc.):** ____________________
- **Phone Number (Back of Card):** ____________________ **Nurse Case Manager:** ____________________

**Secondary Insurance Company:** ____________________

- **Member ID #:** ____________________ **Group #:** ____________________
- **Plan Type (PPO/HMO/etc.):** ____________________
- **Phone Number (Back of Card):** ____________________ **Nurse Case Manager:** ____________________

**2. EMPLOYMENT & LEAVE (HR):** *Tracking who is paying your salary while you are out.*

- **Human Resources Contact (Work):**
  - **Name:** ____________________ **Phone:** ____________________
  - **Email:** ____________________

- **COBRA Administrator:** *If you leave your job, this is who manages your health insurance continuation.*
  - **Company Name:** ____________________ **Phone:** ____________________
  - **Email:** ____________________

**3. DISABILITY & GOVERNMENT:** The complex paperwork. Keep your case numbers here.

- **Short/Long Term Disability (STD/LTD):**
  - **Carrier Name (e.g., The Hartford, Sedgwick, MetLife):** ____________________
  - **Claim #(s):** ____________________ **Claim Specialist Name:** ____________________
  - **Email:** ____________________ **Phone:** ____________________

- **Social Security Disability (SSDI):**
  - **Local Office Phone:** ____________________
  - **Case Worker Name:** ____________________

- **State Paid Leave (if applicable):**
  - **Login/ID:** ____________________

# Medical Snapshot & Care Team

Keep this page updated as a one-stop reference for your clinical team and essential medical data, ensuring you have the right information ready at every appointment.

**The Patient Basics**

- **Primary Diagnosis:** ____________________
- **Date of Diagnosis:** ____________________
- **Secondary Diagnoses/Complications:** ____________________
- **Hospital MRN #:** ____________________ **Blood Type:** ____________
- **Allergies:** ____________________

**Primary Care Team**

- **Clinic Name:** ____________________
- **Lead Provider:** ____________________ **Physician Assistant (PA):** ____________
- **Clinic Location/Floor:** ____________________
- **Main Clinic Phone:** ____________________ **After-Hours/Urgent:** ____________
- **Transplant/Nurse Coordinator(s):** ____________________

**Secondary Care Team:**

- **Clinic Name:** ____________________
- **Lead Provider:** ____________________ **Physician Assistant (PA):** ____________
- **Clinic Location/Floor:** ____________________
- **Main Clinic Phone:** ____________________ **After-Hours/Urgent:** ____________
- **Nurse Coordinator(s):** ____________________

**Pharmacy & Logistics**

- **Primary Pharmacy:** ____________________ **Phone:** ____________
- **Pharmacy Address:** ____________________
- **Emergency Contact (Name/Number):** ____________________

# Scheduled/Maintenance Meds

Update in pencil as dosages and schedules change.

| MEDICATION | DOSAGE/FREQUENCY/ PURPOSE |
| --- | --- |
| | |
| | |
| | |
| | |
| | |
| | |
| | |
| | |
| | |
| | |
| | |
| | |
| | |
| | |
| | |
| | |

# Scheduled/Maintenance Meds

Update in pencil as dosages and schedules change.

**MEDICATION** **DOSAGE/FREQUENCY/ PURPOSE**

# PRN / As-Needed Meds & Supplements

Update in pencil as dosages and schedules change.

| MEDICATION | DOSAGE/FREQUENCY/ PURPOSE |
| --- | --- |
| | |
| | |
| | |
| | |
| | |
| | |
| | |
| | |
| | |
| | |
| | |
| | |
| | |
| | |
| | |
| | |

## Life Outside the Hospital

When you are at the hospital, life at home doesn't stop. Use this page to organize your "village" so you can focus on your health and healing.

### Home & Pet Care

- **House Check /Mail & Trash:** ________________
- **Pet Sitter(s):** ________________
- **Veterinarian:** ________________

### Community & Financial Support

- **Community / Church Liaison(s):** ________________
- **Meal Train Coordinator(s):** ________________
- **Fundraising / Financial Coordinator:** ________________
- **Fundraising Link(s):** ________________

### Hospital Mail & Packages

Most hospitals have mailrooms that deliver directly to your room. You can often have Amazon packages and family care packages sent straight to you so you don't have to pack everything at once. Ask your nurse about unit-specific rules for flowers or certain deliveries.

- **Hospital Name:** ________________
- **Mailing Address:** ________________
- **Patient Name & Room Number:** ________________

### School & Family Logistics (If Applicable)

- **School Name(s):** ________________
- **Principal / Main Office:** ________________
- **School Nurse:** ________________ **Teacher(s):** ________________
- **School Counselor/ 504/IEP Coordinator:** ________________
- **Child Life Specialist:** ________________ **Hospital Social Worker:** ________________
- **Childcare / Sibling Support:** ________________

# Important Medical Terms

Knowledge is power. Understanding these terms will help you decode the jargon, ask better questions, and advocate for the care you need. For specialized terms related to Oncology and Hematology, please refer to the next page.

- **Vitals:** The “Big Four” Vitals: These are checked to monitor your basic stability: Heart Rate (pulse), Blood Pressure, Temperature (checking for infection), and Oxygen (the clip on your finger).
- **Glucose (Blood Sugar):** This is often checked with a “finger stick” test. Even if you aren’t diabetic, steroids and stress can cause increased glucose levels.
- **Electrolytes:** These are essential minerals monitored through blood work: Potassium, Magnesium, Phosphorus, and Calcium. If levels are low, you may be given IV or Oral Replacements (pills, liquids, or drips).
- **Baseline:** What is “normal” for you. Medical teams look for changes from your baseline rather than just a single high or low number.
- **Inpatient vs. Outpatient:** Inpatient means you are staying in the hospital overnight; Outpatient means you receive treatment at a clinic and go home (or to a hotel/house) afterward.
- **Rounding:** The time (usually in the morning) when the entire medical team (Attending, Residents, Pharmacist, etc.) visits your room to discuss your plan for the day.
- **P.R.N. (Pro Re Nata):** A Latin term for “As Needed.” If a medicine is PRN (like for nausea or pain), the nurse won’t give it automatically—you have to ask for it.
- **N.P.O. (Nil Per Os):** Means “Nothing by Mouth.” Usually ordered before a surgery or procedure. No food, no water, no gum.
- **I’s and O’s (Inputs and Outputs):** A hospital task where the team tracks every ounce of fluid you drink and every ounce that leaves your body.
- **PICC Line:** This is a long, thin tube inserted into a vein in your arm and threaded to your heart. It is often used for shorter-term treatments for infusions and blood draws.
- **Trifusion Catheter:** A specialized central line tunneled under the skin of your chest that splits into three separate tubes (lumens), allowing the team to give different treatments simultaneously without them mixing before they reach your heart.
- **Infusion: The “Drip.”** This is just the medical word for receiving your meds (like chemo or fluids) through your PICC Line or IV.
- **Prophylaxis:** The “Shield.” These are meds you take before you feel sick (like anti-nausea or anti-fungals) to prevent a problem before it starts.

# Oncology/Hematology Terms

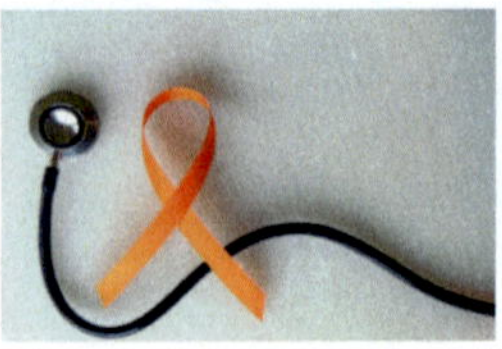

- **WBC (White Blood Cells):** Your overall "Immune Army" that fights off bacteria, viruses, and other foreign invaders.
- **ANC (Absolute Neutrophil Count):** Your "Special Forces"—the specific part of your WBCs most responsible for fighting bacterial infections.
- **HGB (Hemoglobin):** Your "Oxygen Tank"—the protein in red blood cells that carries energy & oxygen to your body (if low, you feel tired/short of breath).
- **Platelets:** Your "Band-Aids"—the tiny cells that stick together to clot your blood and stop you from bruising or bleeding.
- **Cryo (Cryoprecipitate):** This is a specialized blood product that contains a high concentration of Fibrinogen (the "glue" that helps blood clot). It's often given if you are bleeding or if your protein levels are too low to help your platelets do their job.
- **Thrombocytopenia:** The term for a low platelet count.
- **Pancytopenia:** This occurs when White Cells, Red Cells, and Platelets are low at the same time. This usually is due to treatment.
- **Lymphocytes:** These are the white blood cells that specifically target viruses and respiratory infections (like the flu, COVID-19, or pneumonia).
- **Nadir:** The lowest point your blood counts will hit after treatment.
- **Neutropenic:** When your ANC is low, meaning you are at high risk for infection.
- **Blood Transfusion Triggers:** Most hospitals use general benchmarks for transfusions—often around 7 for Hemoglobin and 10–20 for Platelets. Your 'trigger' number may be higher or lower depending on your symptoms, fever, or upcoming procedures. Ask your team: "What is my personal transfusion threshold?"
- **Biopsy / Pathology:** The "Under the Microscope." The biopsy is the procedure to take a sample (e.g., tissue/bone marrow/cerebral spinal fluid 'CSF') and Pathology is the lab report that gives the final, official name of your diagnosis or disease status.
- **Cytogenetics / Molecular Testing:** This is the deep-dive testing they do on your cells to see if there are specific mutations that a "Targeted Therapy" can treat.
- **Mucositis:** Soreness or inflammation in the mouth/throat caused by treatment.
- **TPN (Total Parenteral (IV) Nutrition):** This is a nutrient-rich liquid given directly through your PICC/Trifusion Catheter to provide full nutrition when you can't eat, which is especially helpful if Mucositis makes swallowing too painful.
- **PCA (Patient-Controlled Analgesia):** The "Pain Button"- A computerized pump that lets you safely self-administer pain medicine through your IV for immediate relief.

## Who's Who: Your Hospital Village

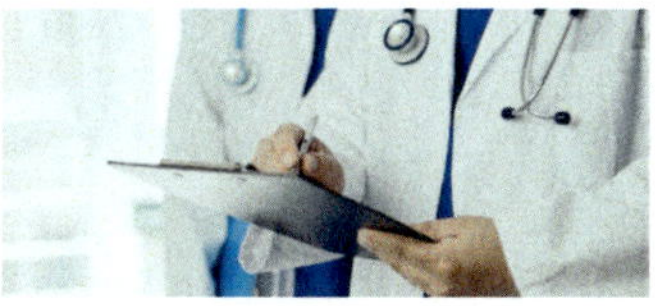

- **Your Primary Oncologist:** The "Long-Term Architect." This is "your" doctor—the one you see in the outpatient clinic. They design the overall treatment map (the big picture). While they communicate with the hospital team, they might not be the one standing at your bedside every morning.

- **The Attending Physician:** The "Captain of the Week." This is the senior doctor in charge of your care while you are in the hospital. They make the final decisions on rounds.
  Note: In teaching hospitals, the Attending often rotates (swaps out) every week, so you may have a different "Captain" on Monday than you did on Friday.

- **Nurse Practitioner (NP) / Physician Assistant (PA):** The "Co-Pilots." These are highly trained medical professionals who work alongside your Attending. They can diagnose, treat, prescribe medication, and discharge you. Because they often stay on the unit longer than rotating residents, they provide crucial continuity and are often faster to respond to needs during the day.

- **Fellows and Residents:** The "Boots on the Ground." Licensed doctors in training who manage your day-to-day medical needs.

- **Your Bedside Nurse (RN):** Your "MVP." Usually one for Day Shift and one for Night Shift. They are your primary point of contact for everything.

- **The Charge Nurse:** The "Floor Manager." They oversee all the nurses on the shift and handle any big-picture logistical issues on the unit.

- **Medical Assistant (MA) / Patient Care Assistant (PCA):** The "Helping Hands." They assist with vitals, mobility, and basic needs.

- **The Clinical Pharmacist:** The "Safety Guard." They check medication dosages and drug interactions.

- **Nurse Case Manager / Social Worker:** Your "Logistics Experts." They bridge the gap between the hospital and the "real world"—handling insurance, FMLA paperwork, and discharge planning.

- **The Transplant Coordinator:** While the doctor is the "Captain," the Transplant Coordinator (usually an RN) is your "Air Traffic Controller" who makes sure everything is in order for your transplant.

- **Dietitian: The "Fuel Expert."** They help manage your nutrition, especially if you are experiencing nausea or have strict dietary requirements.

- **Physical & Occupational Therapy (PT/OT):** The "Mobility Squad." They focus on keeping your body moving to prevent muscle loss and complications (like pneumonia) so you are physically ready for discharge.

- **Medical Scribe:** They record and document what was said in the appointment.

# Care Team Connections

Use this space to keep track of the many hands helping you—from the medical team to the support staff. Writing a personal detail about your team helps strengthen your bond, making your care feel more like a partnership.

| NAME | ROLE | FUN FACT/PERSONAL CONNECTION |
|---|---|---|
| *E.g., Sarah* | *Day Nurse* | *Loves watching the Office & has a pug* |
| | | |
| | | |
| | | |
| | | |
| | | |
| | | |
| | | |
| | | |
| | | |
| | | |
| | | |
| | | |
| | | |

# Care Team Connections

Behind every recovery is a team of humans. Lean on their expertise, learn their stories, and let them help you carry the load.

| NAME | ROLE | FUN FACT/PERSONAL CONNECTION |
| --- | --- | --- |
| | | |
| | | |
| | | |
| | | |
| | | |
| | | |
| | | |
| | | |
| | | |
| | | |
| | | |
| | | |
| | | |
| | | |

# Care Team Connections

Your care team is more than a list of names; they are your greatest allies. When you connect with each person, you build a bridge to better care.

| NAME | ROLE | FUN FACT/PERSONAL CONNECTION |
|---|---|---|
| | | |
| | | |
| | | |
| | | |
| | | |
| | | |
| | | |
| | | |
| | | |
| | | |
| | | |
| | | |
| | | |
| | | |

# Care Team Connections

Your care team is your village. Learn their names, share your story, and turn providers into partners.

| NAME | ROLE | FUN FACT/PERSONAL CONNECTION |
| --- | --- | --- |

BREATHE
IN.
BREATHE
OUT.

PART 2

# THE SANCTUARY STRATEGY

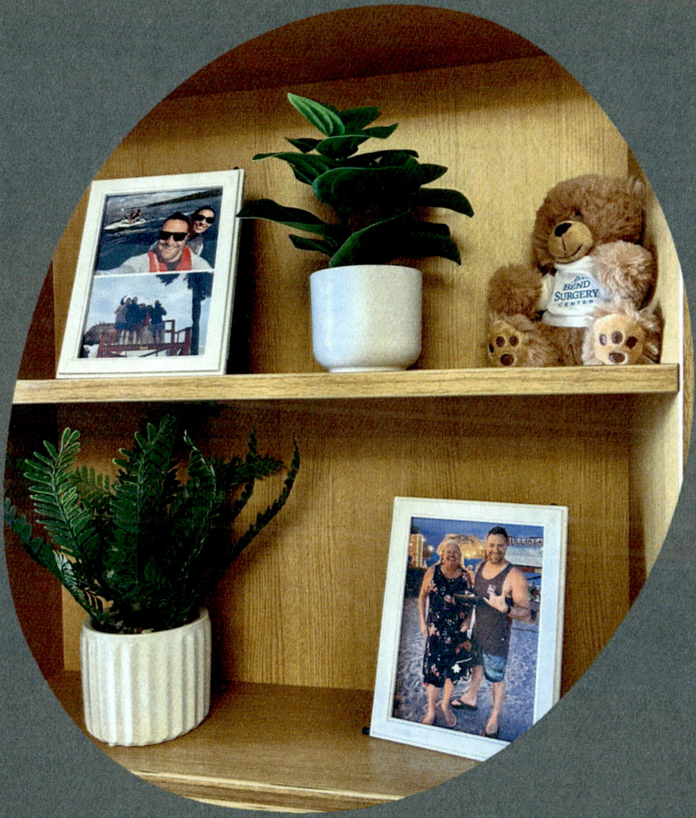

From Packing Your Bags to Creating Your Space

# Environment is Medicine: From Packing Your Bags to Claiming Your Space

We often think of medicine as just treatments and procedures, but the space where you heal is a crucial part of your care. Whether you are checking into a hospital for a month-long stay, heading to a clinic for daily infusions, or navigating recovery on your own couch, your environment is more than just a backdrop. Creating an intentional, comforting space can profoundly shift how you experience your recovery.

In fact, research in environmental psychology demonstrates that our physical surroundings directly impact our physical recovery. A calm, personal space can lower blood pressure, reduce anxiety, and even decrease the perception of pain. While unfamiliar clinical settings can sometimes trigger a stress response, you have the power to change that. By adding familiar, comforting touches, you actively signal to your brain that you are safe.

This isn't just about decoration; it's a tangible tool. Whether you are hanging photos in a hospital ward, taking your own pillow to an outpatient center, or perfectly adjusting the lighting in your own bedroom, you are taking back a piece of your autonomy. This section provides a blueprint for turning any space into a home base where you aren't just a patient—you are a person.

## What's In This Section:

- **The Logistics:** How to pack for the unknown (long-distance and local)
- **The Move-In:** Strategies for organizing your gear and hiding the medical clutter
- **The Setup:** Using sound, light, and visuals to calm your nervous system
- **The Hacks:** Simple ways to connect, like leaving a candy bowl by your door for your care team (pictured right)

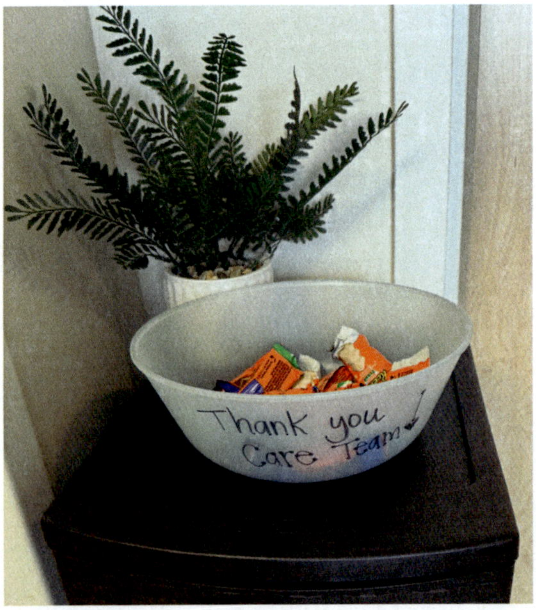

# The Departure: Packing for Your Treatment

We have walked two very different roads, and we know that "packing" looks different for everyone. Regardless of the distance, the goal is the same: Bring the anchors of your life with you.

- **The Long Haul:** For Thomas' leukemia treatment, we drove 3.5 hours to a new city, leaving our home behind for months. We had to pack like we were moving into a dorm room.
- **The Local Treatment:** For Thomas' mom's pancreatic cancer, treatment was close to home. The packing was lighter, focused on infusion appointments and short stays.

## Don't Worry About Forgetting Things

We have spent over 80 nights sleeping in hospital rooms. We did not have a perfect system on Night 1. In fact, we were still refining our packing list and discovering new tips on Night 80! You do not need to pack 100% of your life on Day 1. Most hospitals have a mailroom that delivers packages directly to patient rooms. We had Amazon boxes arriving frequently with needed items. Family and friends were also eager to bring items from home when they came to visit. Focus on the essentials for the first 48 hours, and gather the rest as you go.

### Tips for Caregivers Spending Time in the Hospital

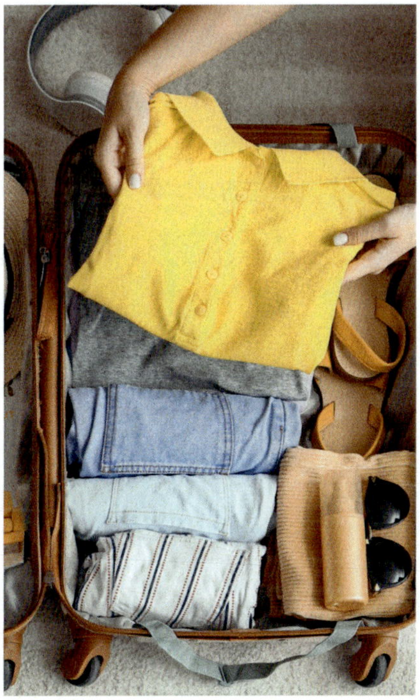

- **Wear Comfortable Shoes**: You will be running errands, getting ice, and walking the halls.
- **Bring Your Own Charger**: A dedicated 10-foot charging cord for your phone is essential.
- **Use Noise-Canceling Headphones**: The hospital is full of beeps and alarms. These are a lifesaver for sleep or if you need to work remotely—I was even able to take Zoom calls right in the hospital room.
- **Pack Warm Clothes:** Hospital temperatures are unpredictable—freezing in the hallway, sweating in the room. Bring a zip-up hoodie or cardigan so you can adjust instantly without changing your whole outfit.
- **Stash Shelf-Stable Snacks:** Keep a supply of protein bars, nuts, and other snacks for when you need fuel.

# Making Your Space a Sanctuary

Transforming a sterile hospital room into a comforting sanctuary was vital for us. We sought to reclaim control and infuse our space with familiar warmth, making it feel like home, not just a medical facility. We achieved this by personalizing it with family photos, soft throw blankets and pillows, and motivational posters. We added fake plants for greenery and celebrated holidays with seasonal decorations, from pumpkins for Halloween to festive trees for Christmas.

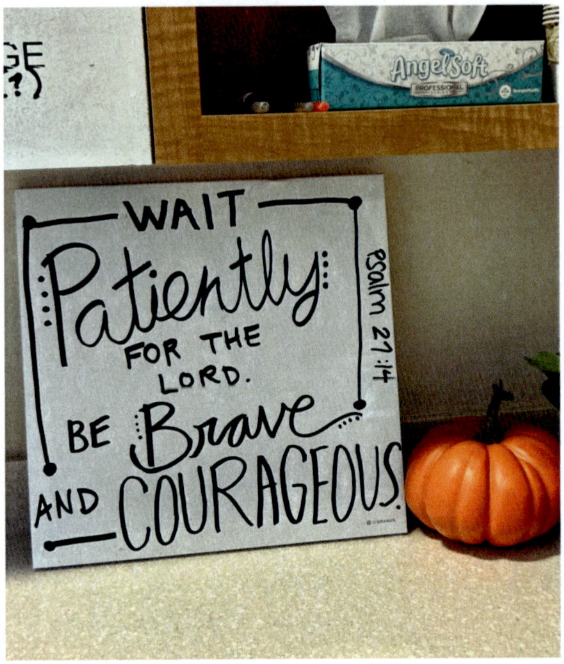


To keep our spirits anchored, I also brought a mini-whiteboard (right) as a daily touchstone, writing a new encouraging Bible verse on it every morning to serve as a constant reminder of hope and strength found in our faith.

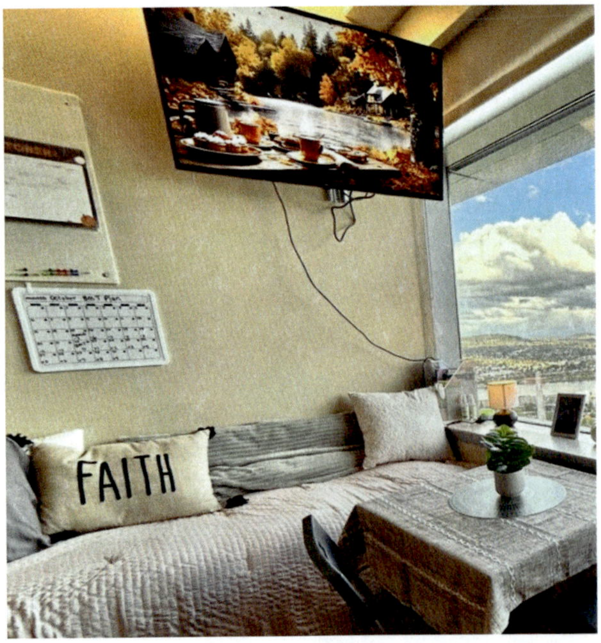


Our efforts paid off; doctors and nurses often commented on how cozy and calming our room felt, even saying they wanted to relax there. We always played soft music—often paired with nature scenes with gentle sounds or peaceful worship music that kept us spiritually grounded. Plus, a small dish of chocolates by the door was always appreciated by our care team. These simple touches profoundly impacted our daily outlook and well-being, proving that a little bit of home goes a long way in healing. We hope you can find peace and comfort in personalizing your space, as these items made a world of difference for us.

# Setting Up Your Hospital Room: Move-In Checklist

Follow these steps to set up and transform your hospital room into a healing space. Watch our Hospital Room Set Up video to see the steps in action!

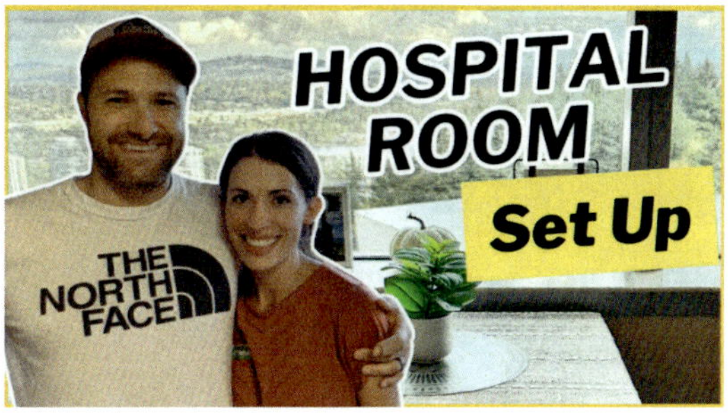


Video Link

**STEP 1: Eliminate the Luggage (The Foundation)**

- Living out of a suitcase signals to your brain that you are in transit or waiting. Unpack your clothes and toiletries directly into the hospital drawers and closets. We brought in a plastic organizer for more space.
- Once empty, stash your bags under the sink, behind the trash cans, or in the bottom of the closet.
- Hang up comfortable clothes. Thomas wore his own T-shirts and athletic pants. This meant Lindsey did laundry, but it was worth it!

**STEP 2: Soften the Edges (The Atmosphere)**

- Place your fake plants on the window sill or counters. This adds instant life and color to the room. (Real plants aren't allowed on certain hospital floors).
- Use blue painter's tape or sticky tack to hang motivational posters and family photos where the patient can see them from the bed.
- The Chocolate Bowl: Place a bowl of treats near the door and write "Thank you care team" on the bowl. This invites the staff to pause and smile when they enter.

**STEP 3: The Tech Command Center (The Connection)**

- Ask your nurse for the Hospital Guest Wi-Fi password and get connected.
- Locate the outlets and plug in chargers. They are often behind the bed.
- Connect your Streaming Device to the hospital TV using your 8-foot HDMI cord if possible. (Check the side or back of the TV for the HDMI port).
- Set up the White Noise Machine near the door to block hallway noise and pair your Bluetooth Speaker for music.

# Hospital Packing List

## Personal Care

- ○ Comfortable Clothes
- ○ Robe/Warm Sweatshirt
- ○ Slippers (non-slip soles)
- ○ Shower Shoes
- ○ Shower Caddy
- ○ Waterproof PICC Sleeve
- ○ PICC Access Sweatshirt
- ○ Glasses (if you wear them)
- ○ Soft Toothbrush + Paste
- ○ Deodorant
- ○ Shampoo + Conditioner
- ○ Sleep Eye Mask

## Room Decor & Living

- ○ Books/Journals/Bible
- ○ Motivational Wall Art
- ○ Photos/ Picture Frames
- ○ Painter's Tape/Sticky Tack
- ○ Wall Calendar
- ○ Decorative Pillow
- ○ Small Folding Table and Chairs (if space)
- ○ Plastic Organizer with Drawers for storage (if space)
- ○ Table Cloth
- ○ Fake Plants
- ○ Games
- ○ Transplant/medical book
- ○ Binder for important papers

## Comfort & Bedding

- ○ Insulated Water Bottle
- ○ Neck fan & Ice Beanie (for chemo hot flashes)
- ○ Peppermint Essential Oil Roller (for Nausea)
- ○ Chemo Headwear
- ○ Wisdom Teeth Ice Pack Wrap (for mucositis)
- ○ Mattress Topper Twin XL
- ○ Mattress Pad for Caregiver
- ○ Cooling Comfort Blanket
- ○ Your Own Pillow
- ○ Snacks & Condiments

## Tech Essentials

- ○ Streaming Device (Apple TV, Roku, Fire Stick, etc.)
- ○ 8ft HDMI Cord (needed for your streaming device)
- ○ Chargers (extra-long cords)
- ○ Laptop/Tablet
- ○ Bluetooth Speaker
- ○ White Noise Machine

## Other

- ○ ..............................................................
- ○ ..............................................................
- ○ ..............................................................

Product Links

# Sanctuary Recommendations

Your environment profoundly impacts your daily outlook. These items are designed to bridge the gap between 'medical facility' and 'home,' helping to boost your mood, maintain normalcy, and provide much-needed sensory comfort during long stays.

Product Links

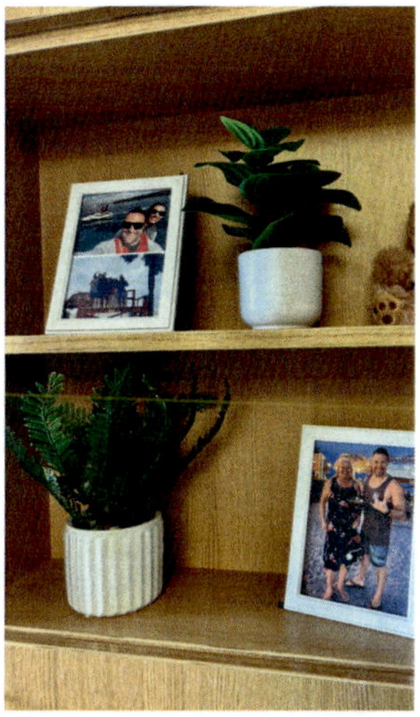

- **Potted Fake Plants**: A touch of greenery can brighten any room and requires no upkeep.
- **Motivational Wall Quotes**: Bring inspiring messages directly to your line of sight.
- **Wall Calendar**: Keep track of your days and celebrate reaching medical milestones.
- **Picture Frames**: Fill with photos of loved ones or cherished memories to bring familiarity and joy.
- **White Noise Machine**: Create a calming sound environment for better rest or focus.
- **Apple TV**: Or other streaming device for entertainment and a sense of normalcy during long stays.
- **HDMI Cord (8 Foot)**: To connect your streaming device to the hospital room tv.
- **Bluetooth Speaker**: To play music in your room.
- **Decorative Pillow**: A cozy and comforting item to personalize your space and bring a sense of home.

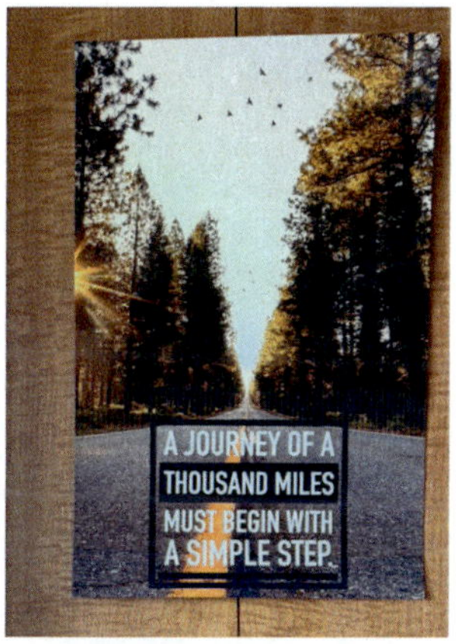


- **Table and 2 Folding Chairs & Chair Pad**: We were fortunate to have enough space in our hospital room for a small, foldable table and chair set we found at IKEA. This was a complete game-changer for us—it gave us a dedicated spot for meals, working on puzzles, and staying organized. Having a 'normal' surface away from the medical bed made the room feel more functional and less like a clinical facility. Always ask your hospital staff before bringing in furniture or electronics to ensure they are cleared for your specific unit.

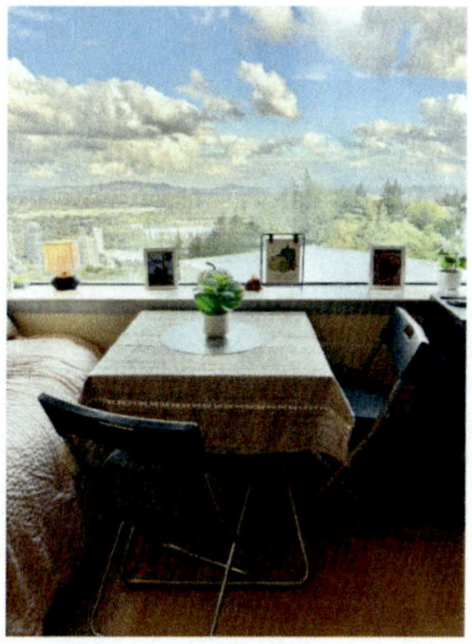

- **Small Tablecloth**: A simple way to hide a cold, clinical surface and make a hospital table feel like your dining room at home. We found it made our "date night" meals feel much more normal and special.

I CAN DO
HARD
THINGS.

PART 3

# THE MINDSET & BODY TOOLKIT

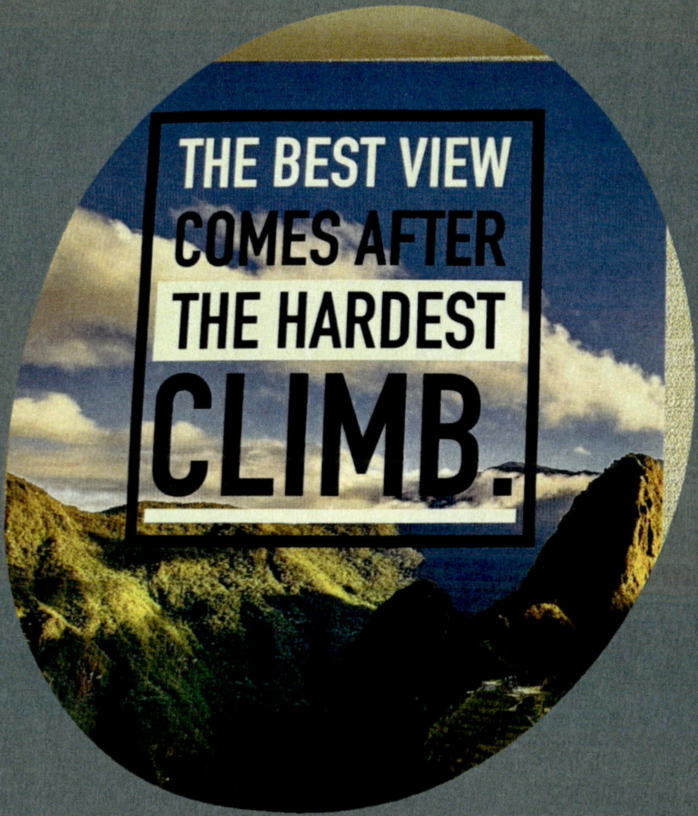


## Essential Strategies for the Marathon of Treatment

# Thriving Through Treatment: A Holistic Approach

## Your Holistic Toolkit

A health journey is as much a mental and emotional experience as it is a physical one. We discovered that true healing happens when you support the whole person—body, mind, and spirit. This section is your "Thrive Kit." It is a curated collection of our favorite discoveries designed to bring you ease, comfort, and confidence.

## Why We Combined Body & Mind

Physical comfort and mental resilience go hand-in-hand. When your body is uncomfortable—whether you are cold, hot, or surrounded by harsh lighting—your brain stays in "Fight or Flight" mode, flooding your system with stress hormones like cortisol. Prioritizing physical comfort sends a biological signal to your brain that you are safe.

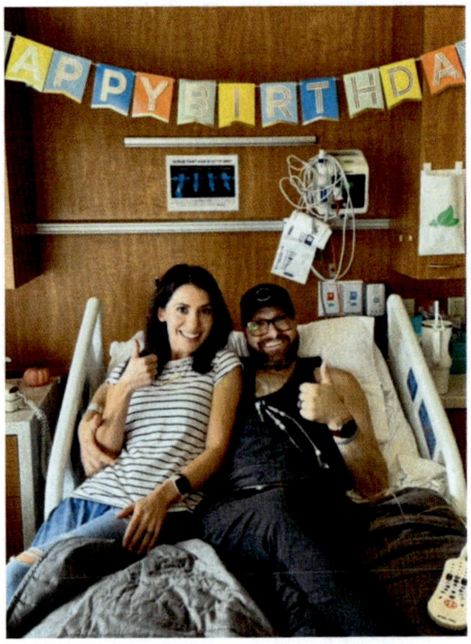

However, the reverse is also true! Your emotional well-being profoundly impacts your physical recovery. Navigating the heavy emotions of treatment, staying connected to your loved ones, and actively processing grief helps flip the switch to your Parasympathetic Nervous System (the "Rest and Digest" state). By deeply supporting your mind and spirit, you allow your body to focus all of its energy on healing.

## What's In This Section:

- **Physical Comforts:** Items to streamline your routine and bring physical ease
- **Mental Resilience:** Brain-backed strategies to process heavy emotions
- **Ways to Boost Your Mood:** A quick-reference guide to cultivating joy
- **Care Partner Support:** Essential tips to ensure the caregiver stays supported
- **Staying Connected as a Couple:** Tools to nurture your relationship
- **Navigating Treatment with Kids:** Strategies to help children feel safe and involved
- **Navigating Grief:** Compassionate guidance for processing complex loss
- **Cultivating Gratitude:** Practical strategies for finding pockets of joy during heavy seasons
- **Hope-Filled Phrases:** Daily reminders to ground your mindset
- **Anchors of Encouragement:** A space to write the quotes, scriptures, or personal thoughts that are most meaningful to you

# Personal Comfort & Self-Care

The physical toll of treatment can be immense, and maintaining personal comfort often falls by the wayside in a medical setting. However, prioritizing self-care —even in small ways—is critical for both physical recovery and mental fortitude. We learned this early on: Thomas' first hospital stay immediately highlighted how notoriously uncomfortable hospital beds can be, leading us to invest in a mattress topper right away. Throughout his treatment, especially with various chemo drugs, Thomas would experience intense hot sweats at different times of the day; having an ice beanie, a cooling blanket, and a fan he wore around his neck proved invaluable for managing these.

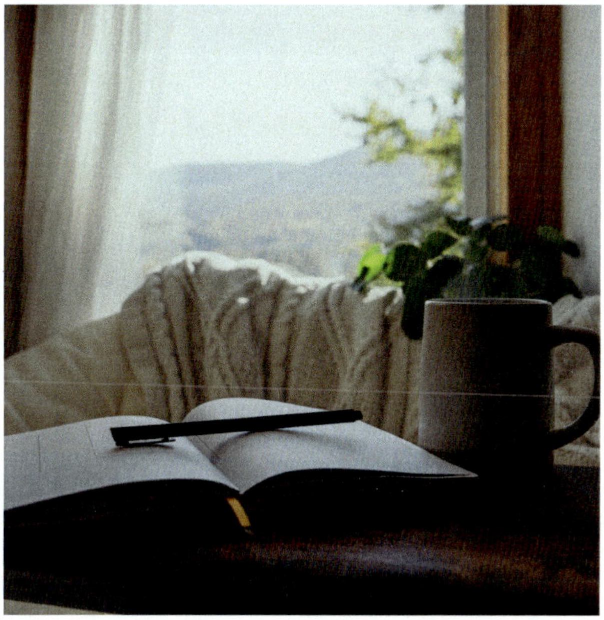

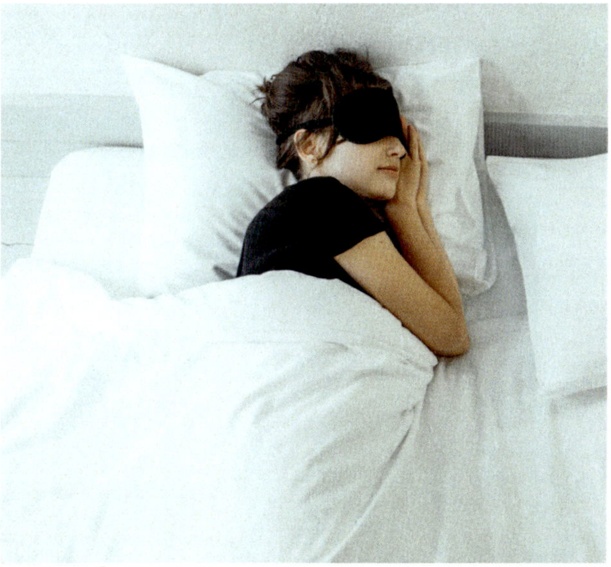

Trying to fall asleep in a bright, noisy hospital room was incredibly difficult for both Thomas and me, so eye masks became an absolute must-have. Beyond managing specific symptoms, sometimes comfort was about maintaining a sense of normalcy and dignity. Wearing robes in the morning, for instance, made us feel like we were at a fancy hotel, even when we were still very much in a hospital room. And later, after the transplant, we quickly discovered that dry mouth and dry eye were very real, persistent side effects, making those specific products essential for daily relief. These items helped us proactively manage discomforts and maintain a sense of personal well-being.

# Personal Comfort Recommendations

These items were the "game-changers" for Thomas' comfort, both during his long hospital stays and throughout his recovery at home.

Product Links

**Please Note**: Every hospital has different rules regarding outside items. Please check with your nursing team before bringing these in, specifically regarding electrical items (like fans), scents (essential oils), or mattress toppers to ensure they meet your unit's safety and infection control standards.

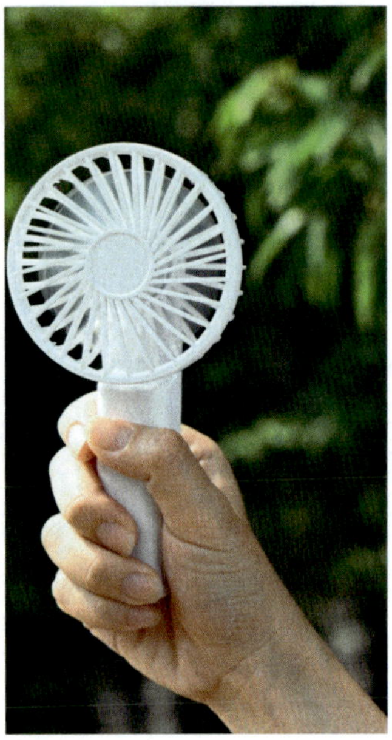

- **Mattress Topper Twin XL Size**: Hospital beds can be notoriously uncomfortable; this made a huge difference for Thomas. Note: We purchased a new, clean topper for each hospital stay to ensure we were adhering to strict infection control and keeping his environment as sterile as possible.
- **Cooling Comfort Blanket**: Essential for managing temperature fluctuations and finding a soft spot.
- **Ice Beanie**: Great for managing headaches, fevers, or just cooling down.
- **Battery Powered Neck Fan**: For personal airflow and comfort when you need it most.
- **Sleep Eye Mask**: Block out light for deeper, more restful sleep.
- **Rubber Sole Slippers**: Easy to slip on for comfort around the room.
- **Comfortable Robe**: A familiar, comfortable robe can make a hospital stay feel more like home.
- **Shower Shoes**: For safety and comfort in hospital showers.
- **Biotene Moisturizing Mouth Spray / XyliMelts for Dry Mouth Night Time**: Essential for managing dry mouth, a common side effect of treatment/GVHD.
- **Preservative-Free Eye Drops**: Essential for lubricating dry eyes, a common symptom of GVHD.
- **Double or Single Leg Elevation Pillow**: For comfort, circulation, and reducing swelling.
- **Aromatherapy for Nausea**: Gentle, natural relief for common treatment side effects.
- **Essential Oils**: Use calming scents like lavender for relaxation and scents like peppermint for nausea relief.

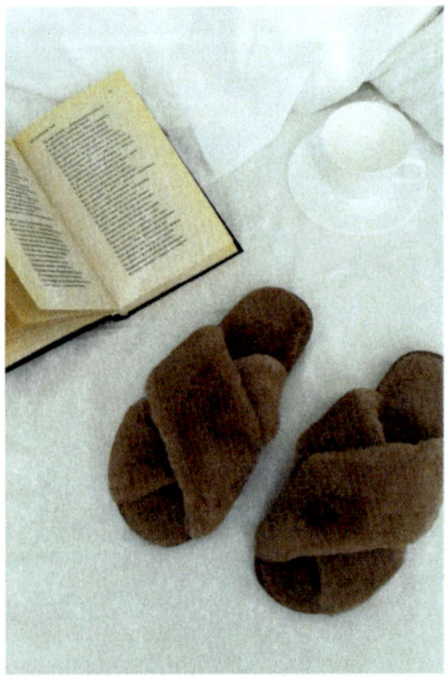

# Meeting Medical Needs

The world of medical treatment can feel overwhelmingly complex and deeply out of your control. From deciphering medical jargon to enduring endless procedures and managing difficult side effects, it's easy to feel adrift. That's why we found it so empowering to regain a sense of practical control and actively adapt to the unique demands of Thomas' medical journey. These items aren't just conveniences; they're strategic tools designed to streamline daily life in the hospital and beyond. They offer solutions for everything from ensuring your PICC line doesn't get wet in the shower and protecting a vulnerable immune system with essential masks, to meticulously managing complex medication schedules to reduce anxiety and ensure adherence.

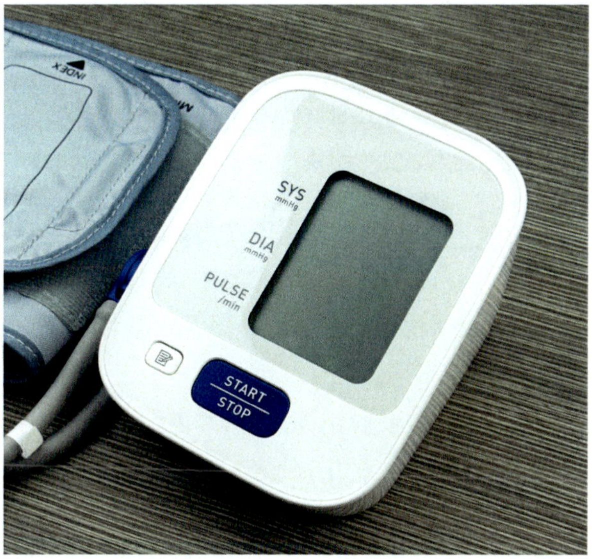


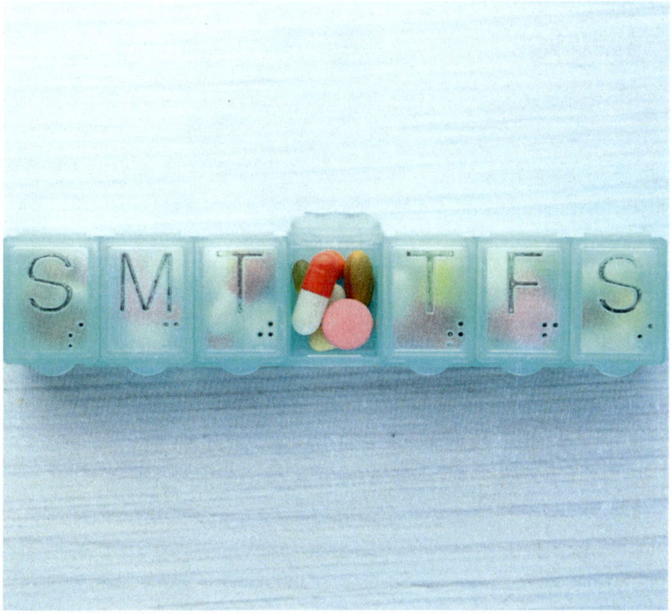


Moreover, they help in adapting to new physical realities, whether it's dealing with reduced mobility and fatigue or coping with increased photosensitivity that can accompany conditions like GVHD. Ultimately, these practical tools aim to make the day-to-day process smoother, less stressful, and a little more manageable. Many of these solutions, including the PICC line shower cover, were even recommended directly by Thomas' nurses and transplant doctor. Looking back, we only wish we'd discovered these essential tools earlier in our medical journey.

**A Note on Medical Gear:**

While these tools were vital to our success, every patient and hospital protocol is different. Please consult your attending physician or nursing team before using any medical gear, supplements, or appliances to ensure they are safe for your specific treatment plan.

# Recommended Support Items

The following items were essential parts of our daily care kit as recommended by our medical team.
**Please Note:** Always consult your specific doctor or nursing lead before using these items, as protocols can change based on your individual treatment plan.

Product Links

- **Blood Pressure Monitor**: Helpful for tracking your readings once you've been discharged from the hospital.
- **Wisdom Teeth Syringe**: Helpful for gentle oral care, especially with mouth sores.
- **Reusable Waterproof Picc Line Sleeve Cover For Upper Arm**: Keep your PICC line safe and dry during showers.
- **KN95 Face Mask Pack**: Essential for protecting a compromised immune system and great to give to people who want to visit you in the hospital.
- **Weekly Pill Organizer**: Keep your medications organized and on schedule.
- **Walking Cane**: For mobility support when energy levels are low or balance is off.
- **Nighttime Lubricant Eye Ointment Dry eye relief**: For managing dry eyes, a common side effect of certain treatments or GVHD (he uses Systane brand).
- **Heat Eye Compress**: For dry or irritated eyes.
- **Wide Brim Sun Hat with Neck Flap / Sun Protection Hoodie**: Crucial for sun protection, especially when photosensitivity is an issue (e.g., with GVHD).
- **Tank Top**: Simple, comfortable clothing that can be layered (he used Amazon Essentials Men's Tank Top).
- **MEDICAL WEAR PICC Access Sweatshirt / Chemo Port Shirts**: Practical and comfortable clothing designed for easy medical access.
- **Compression Socks**: For circulation and comfort, especially during extended periods of rest.
- **Chemo Headwear**: Soft head coverings during hair loss.

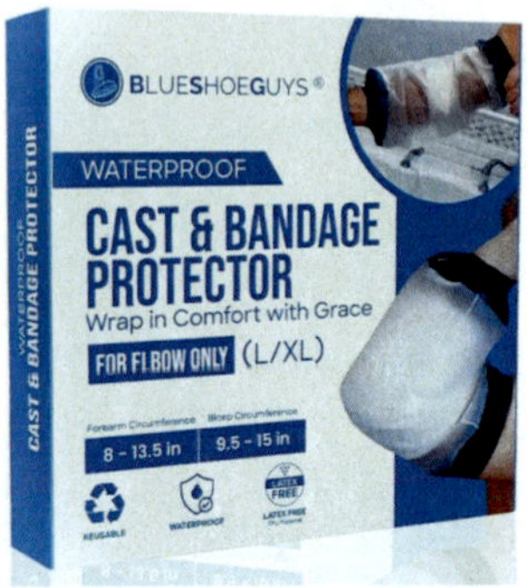


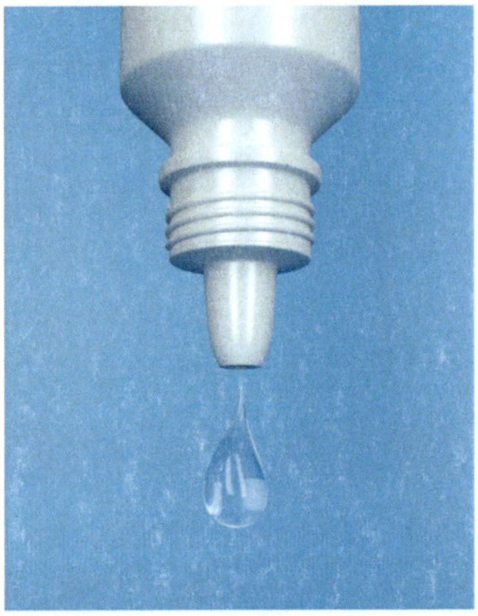

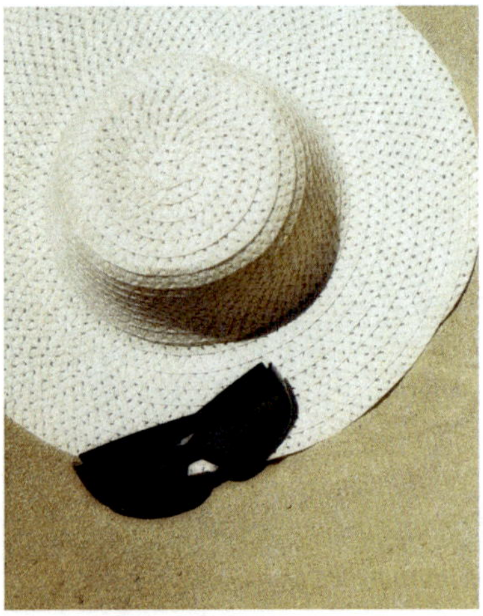

# Infusing Inspiration

Cultivating a positive mindset, finding sources of inspiration, and embracing support are crucial for navigating the ups and downs of any medical journey. These tools are designed to help you practice gratitude, process emotions, stay organized to reduce stress, and find comforting messages of hope. They encourage resilience, reminding you that while you may not control your circumstances, you can cultivate your outlook and draw strength from within and around you.

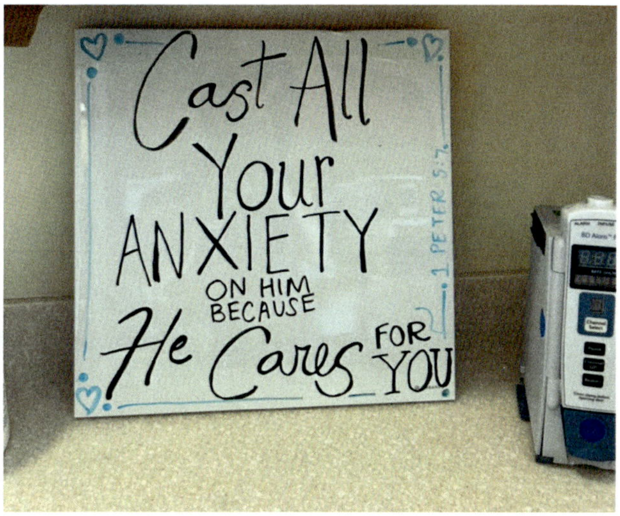


We learned this firsthand, both during Thomas' hospital stays and beyond. We kept a journal every day, writing down what happened and what we were grateful for.

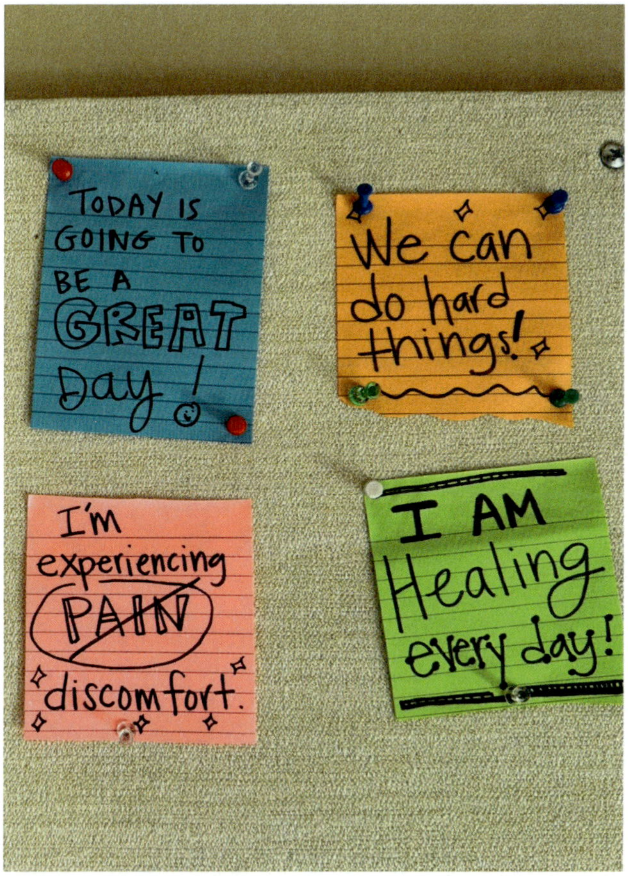


To personalize our space and keep our spirits up, we created a bulletin board on our hospital room wall, filling it with pictures of friends and family, hanging encouraging cards, and posting motivational sticky notes. As we mentioned earlier, we also wrote a new encouraging scripture on our whiteboard daily.

We also created several resources to help us cope, including our "How to Psychologically Cope with Discomfort" page for navigating pain, our "Brain-Backed Ways to Boost Your Mood" page, and a "Day +__" page to track our progress post-transplant, celebrating each small win with a dry-erase marker.

# PSYCHOLOGICALLY *Cope with Discomfort*

## Take calming breaths.

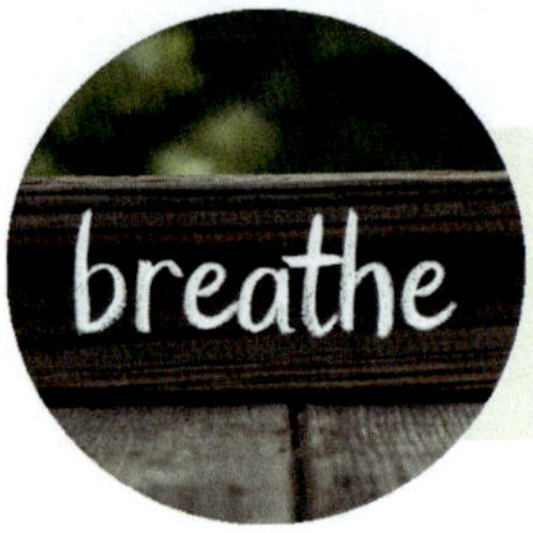


Inhale slowly through your nose, feeling your abdomen expand. Exhale slowly through your mouth or nose, letting your abdomen relax. Repeat.

## Rebrand the idea of pain.

*Replace "I'm in pain" with **"I'm experiencing discomfort."** Discomfort is your body's way of communicating with your brain so you can heal.

## Practice self-compassion.

Tell yourself, "It's okay to feel anxious, worried, and sad. These emotions are normal." Practice holding space for all your feelings and withhold judgment.

## Remember this is temporary.

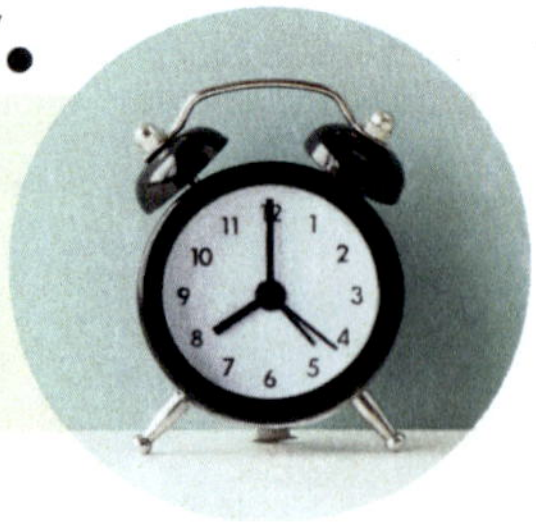

Remind your brain this is temporary. This is a short-term experience. The discomfort will subside.

## Redirect your attention.

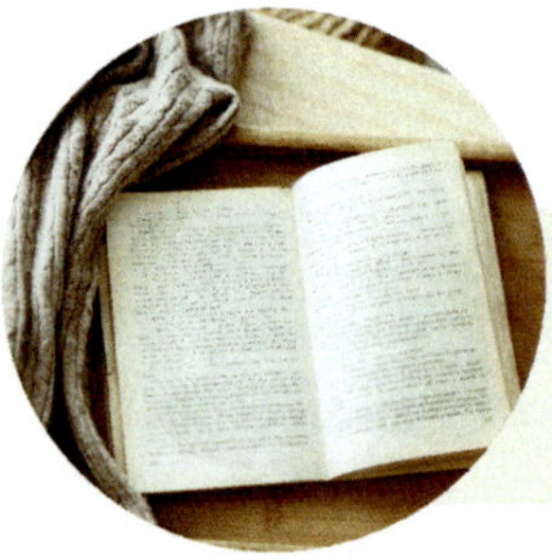

Distract your brain from the discomfort. Call a friend, watch a show with family, read a book, or listen to music or a podcast.

**Always communicate your actual pain levels to your medical team for proper management.*

# BRAIN-BACKED WAYS TO *Boost Your Mood*

## Savor a Snack

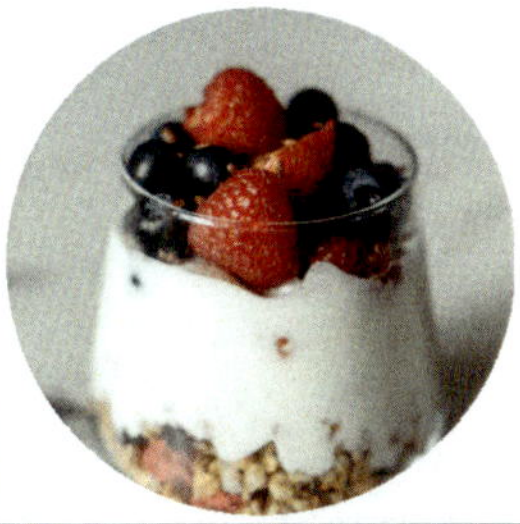

Mindfully enjoy a healthy snack, focusing on the taste, texture, and smell.

## Sunshine Time

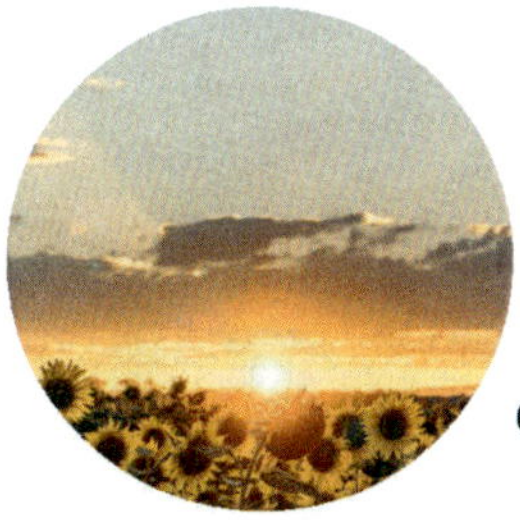

Get bright light: spend time outdoors or use a light therapy box, especially in winter.

## Walk it Out

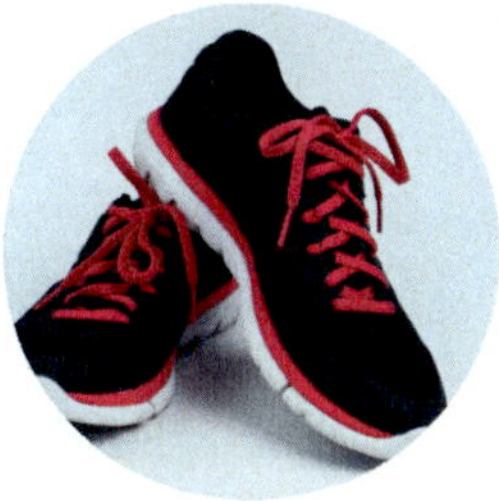

Take a short walk (indoors or out) or try simple movement. Bonus: Invite a friend!

## Sleep Tight

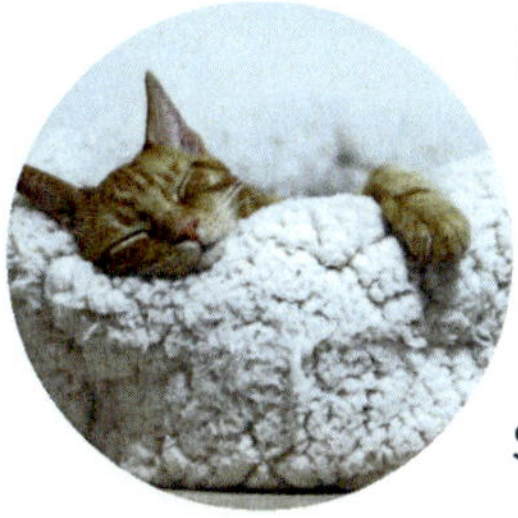

Establish a regular sleep schedule, create a calming bedtime routine, and optimize your sleep environment.

## Future Focus

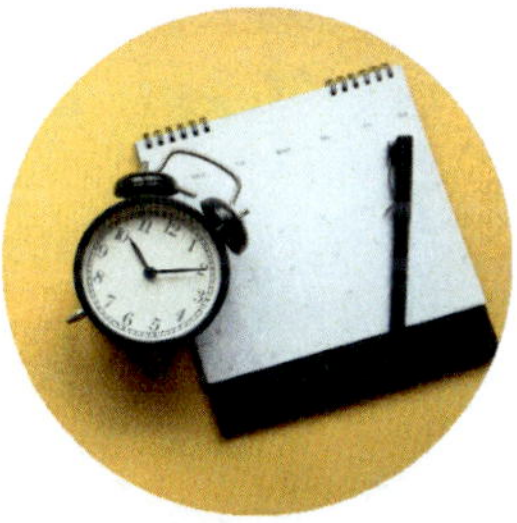

Plan a fun activity, set a small goal, or simply daydream about your future.

## Creative Outlets

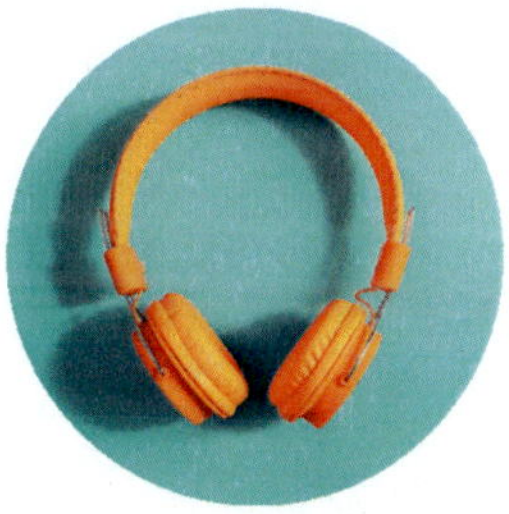

Create a playlist of your favorite uplifting songs, listen to podcasts, or read, write, or draw!

## Connect & Recharge

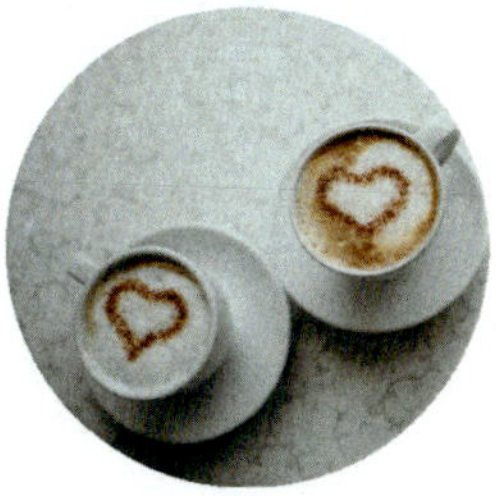

Call or spend time with a friend, family member, or loved one.

## Be Mindful

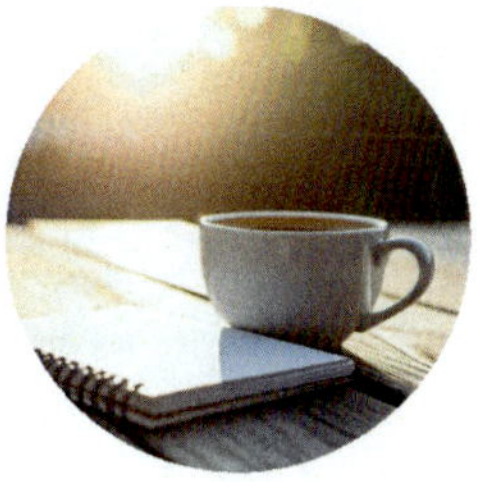

Ground yourself in prayer, meditation, and/or mindfulness. Journal your gratitudes in the back of this book.

# DAY +

**Tip:** To print a fresh copy of this page, scan the QR code on Page 5. You can then place it in a plastic page protector and use a dry erase marker to track your milestones daily!

## Recommended Inspiration & Support Items

Maintaining a positive and organized mindset is a daily practice. These resources helped us anchor our thoughts, stay focused on the "next right thing," and find moments of light during the heavy days.

Product Links

In the photo below, we are wearing our "Faith Over Fear" bracelets—reminders we shared with family and friends in solidarity. You can also see our "Day +" sign on the fridge at the Ronald McDonald House. We originally hoped to be home by Day 100, but we had to stay longer for additional treatment. We kept our milestone sign in a simple page protector and updated it daily with a dry erase marker; it was a small but powerful ritual that reminded us we were still moving forward.

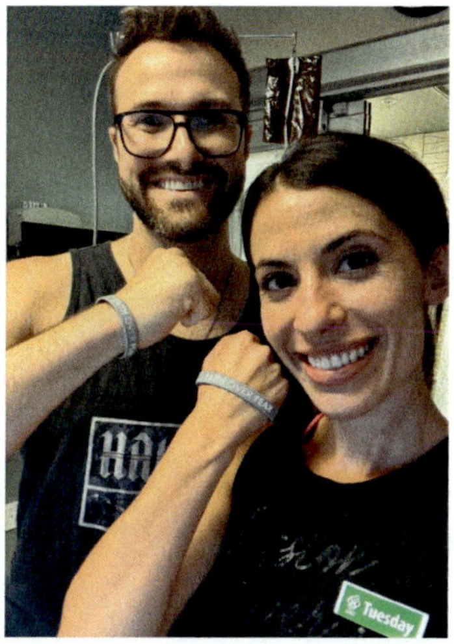

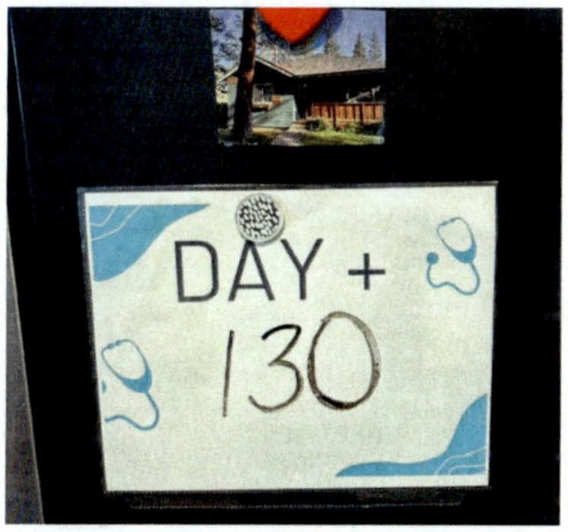


- **The 5-Minute Gratitude Journal**: A quick and easy way to practice gratitude daily.
- **Daily Prayer & Gratitude Journal**: A dedicated space to record thoughts, prayers, and daily gratitudes, helping to process emotions and focus on positive moments.
- **Daily To Do List Notepad**: Helps break down overwhelming tasks into manageable "next right steps."
- **Inspirational Bracelets**: These can serve as a personal reminder of strength and hope, and can also be shared with friends and family as a symbol of unity and support during the journey.
- **Red Blood Cell Plush/White Blood Cell Plush**: A lighthearted way to engage with the science of the body and bring a smile.

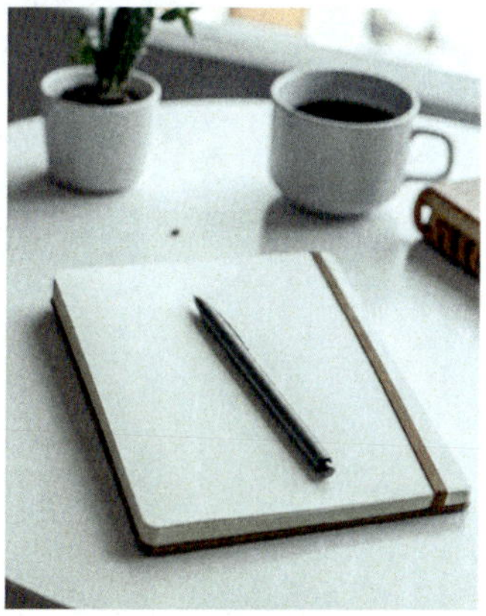

# The Ripple Effect: Healing Together

When a medical crisis hits, it doesn't just impact the patient—it creates a ripple effect that touches every person in their orbit. Roles shift, routines change, and the emotional weight can feel heavy. In the chaos of appointments and treatments, it is incredibly easy to become so focused on physical survival that the emotional needs of the family unit are unintentionally left behind. But true healing requires supporting the entire community.

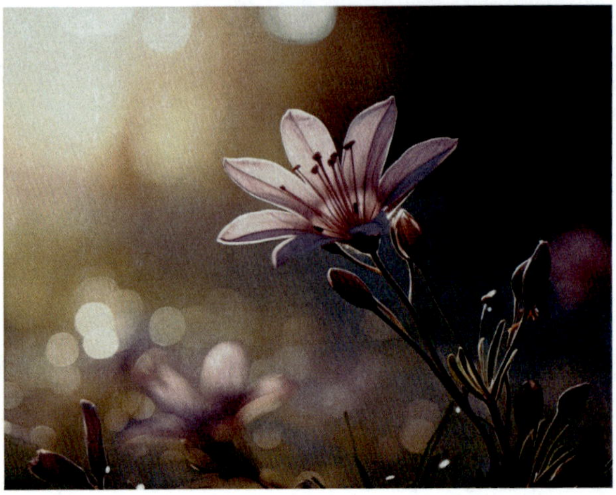

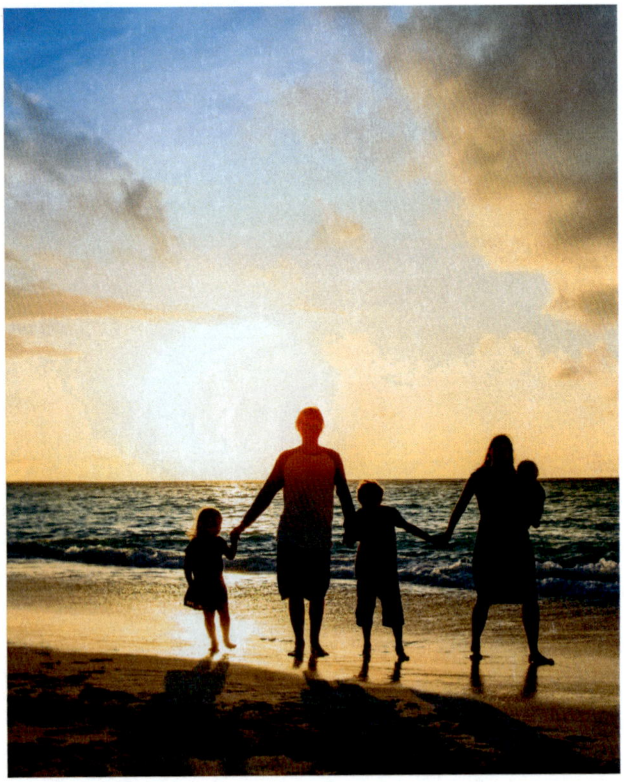

In the following pages, we hold space for the profound, often unspoken relational challenges of a health journey. We will explore how to establish vital boundaries to protect the care partner from burnout, share intentional strategies for staying connected as a couple, and provide tools to help children feel safe, seen, and involved.

Finally, we offer compassionate guidance for navigating the complex layers of grief that accompany a difficult diagnosis. Grief in this season is rarely just about the fear of the future; it is also the immediate mourning of your "normal"—the canceled plans, the shifting of roles, and the life you had before the illness. We will help you hold space for these heavy emotions so you can process them healthily. Your relationships are a vital anchor—this section is designed to protect them.

# Care for the Care Partner

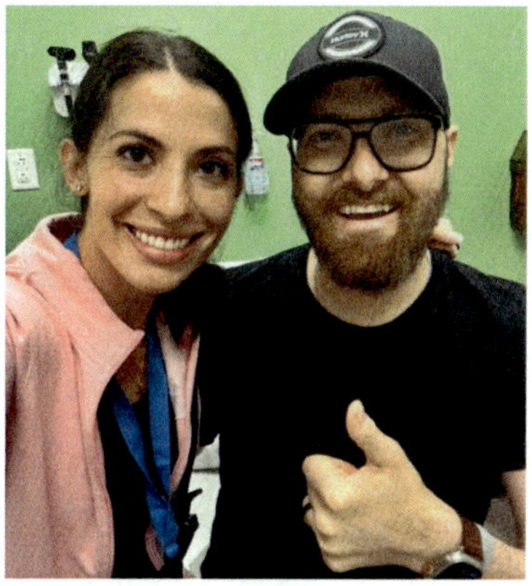

## A Note from Lindsey: The Honor of Showing Up

Serving as the care partner for my husband (through his leukemia and bone marrow transplant) and my mother-in-law (through terminal pancreatic cancer) simultaneously has been challenging and one of the great honors of my life. The past two years taught me a hard truth:
**You cannot pilot the plane if you run out of fuel.**
This page is your permission slip to take care of yourself so you can keep showing up for them.

### 1. The Shift: "Caregiver" vs. "Care Partner"

Words define our reality. While we use the terms "caregiver" and "care partner" interchangeably throughout this guide, we often prefer care partner because it acknowledges a mutual alliance. You aren't just doing for the patient; you are doing with them. You and your loved one are partners in this health journey, tackling decisions, fears, and daily hurdles together as a unified team. Likewise, your loved one can find ways to support you!

### 2. The Best Friend Rule (Self-Compassion)

When the guilt of taking a break creeps in, ask yourself Dr. Kristin Neff's golden question: "Would I treat my best friend this way?" If your best friend was exhausted, would you tell them they were lazy for taking a nap? No! You would tell them to rest. Extend that same grace to yourself.

### 3. Redefine Your "Wins"

In the hospital, productivity looks different. Stop measuring your days by your "normal" standards and start celebrating the micro-wins that keep you human.

- Did you take a shower today?
- Did you step outside to call your mom?
- Did you eat a meal sitting down? Celebrate these wins!

### 4. The "Gift" of Receiving

Asking for help is incredibly difficult. It often challenges our identity as the "strong one" and makes us worry that we are becoming a burden. But here is the truth: Your friends and family likely feel helpless right now. They are watching you struggle and don't know what to do. When you allow someone to help—whether it's mowing your lawn, bringing a meal, or sitting with the patient while you nap—you aren't taking from them. You are giving them the gift of purpose. You are alleviating their helplessness by giving them a tangible way to show their love. Let them in.

### 5. Have Hope

This might be the hardest chapter in your story, but it is not the final chapter. When Thomas started treatment, we grieved the loss of our fertility. But we later discovered a beautiful new path to parenthood through domestic infant adoption. The dreams and plans you once held onto might look different after the hospital, but please hold onto hope—what replaces them might just be more beautiful than you ever imagined.

# The Heart of the Partnership: Staying Connected as a Couple

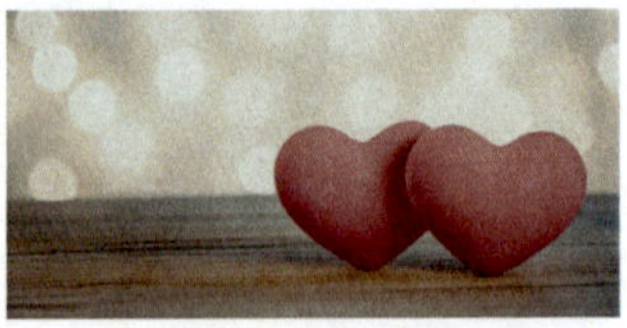

In the storm of treatment, it is easy to slip into the roles of 'Patient' and 'Care Partner' and lose your identity as a couple. This page is a reminder to nurture your marriage as much as your health.

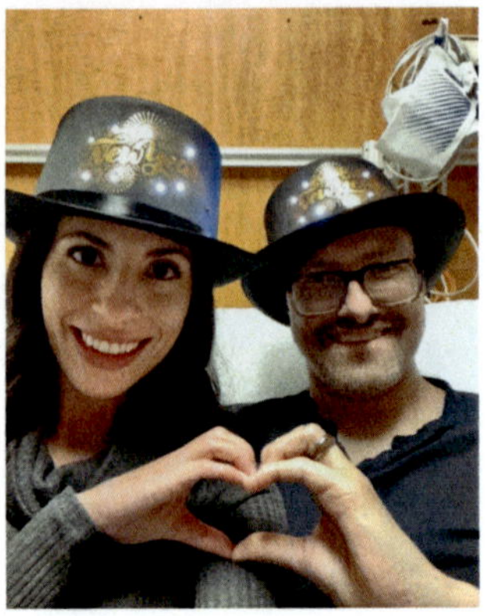

**The Med-Cup Realization**
At one point during Thomas' first hospital stay, Lindsey realized the only physical touch they had shared all day was the passing of a medication cup or a water glass. Don't let your connection become purely clinical. Here are some tips:

- **The 20-Second Hug:** Dr. John Gottman recommends a hug of at least 20 seconds. This releases oxytocin and signals to your nervous system that you are safe in each other's arms.
- **Hold Hands:** In waiting rooms, during difficult consultations, or while walking to appointments—don't let go. It is a silent, powerful anchor of solidarity.
- **Reclaim the Bed:** If the hospital allows, sit together or cuddle in the hospital bed. Reclaiming that physical closeness is powerful medicine for the soul.
- **Remember to Laugh:** Bring the "normal" world inside. Watch a favorite funny show, follow a comedy podcast, or share a private joke. Laughter is the fastest way to lower cortisol.
- **Hospital Date Nights:** Reclaim your time. Dim the lights, order a favorite meal (if allowed), and spend an hour not talking about labs or scans.

**Navigating the Stress Together: This Applies for ALL Relationships!**

Medical stress spikes "fight or flight" hormones. Use these tools to protect your communication:

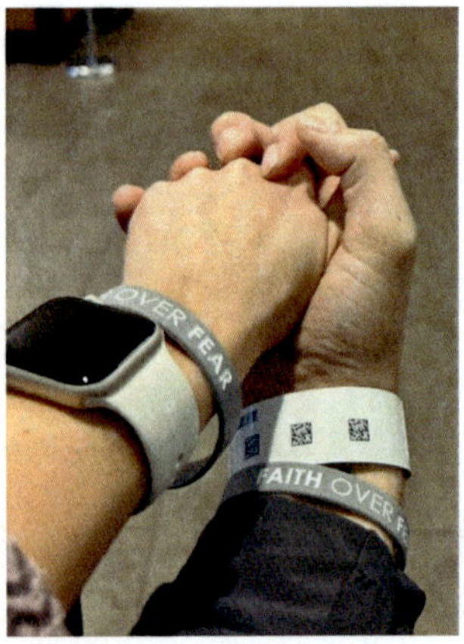


- **Problem-Solve vs. "Feel Felt":** Inspired by Dr. Tina Payne Bryson, clarify what is needed before a heavy conversation. Ask: "Do you want me to help you problem-solve, or do you just need to 'feel felt' right now?"

- **The Pause:** If conflict spikes, pause and ask: Are we "hangry"? Are we exhausted? Give yourselves grace—it's the situation that's the enemy, not each other.

# Navigating Treatment with Kids: The 3 C's

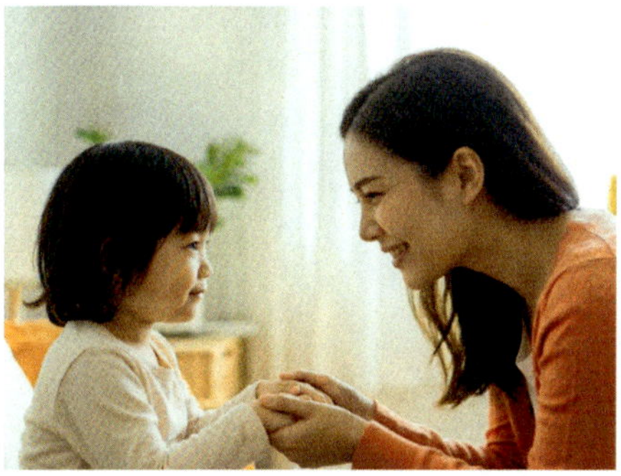

A medical diagnosis affects the entire family, and children often process this stress differently than adults. Based on the PAWsitive Choices Social & Emotional Learning curriculum, you can practice the 3 C's to build emotional regulation during a family health crisis. Scan the QR code on page 5 to access downloadable emotion pictures and videos to help your child identify their feelings and build emotional regulation and problem-solving skills.

## Connect

**Connect:** The hospital environment and changes at home can be intimidating. Normalize this by acknowledging children's feelings and letting them know you are there for them.

- **Validate Emotions:** Remind them it's okay to feel mad, sad, disappointed, or scared.
- **Start the Conversation:** Ask, "How are you feeling?" or "How did that make you feel?"
- **Give Them the Words:** When children aren't able to talk about their feelings, describe what happened for them. (Example: "It makes sense that you feel sad that we can't play outside today. It is hard when our routine changes.")

## Calm

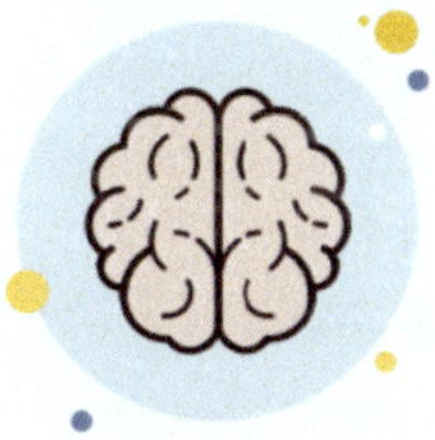

**Calm:** Kids regulate their nervous systems by mirroring their caregivers. Help children regain calm by encouraging them to breathe, take a brain break, or make a different healthy choice.

- **Take a Breath:** Guide them by saying, "Let's take deep breaths" or ask, "What does your brain need?"
- **Step Away:** If the hospital room or a difficult moment becomes too much, step out into the hallway and say, "Let's see if a brain break will help your brain feel in control of your strong feelings."

## Collaborate

**Collaborate:** Medical crises can make kids feel helpless. When they are calm, work together to problem solve.

- **Explore:** Ask, "What were you feeling, thinking, or wanting?"
- **Empower:** While they cannot "fix" the illness, you can empower them to help in other ways by asking, "How can you fix the problem and make things better?"
- **Give Them a Job:** Let them be in charge of picking out hospital room decorations, bringing a favorite stuffed animal for comfort, or choosing the family movie for the night.

# Navigating Grief

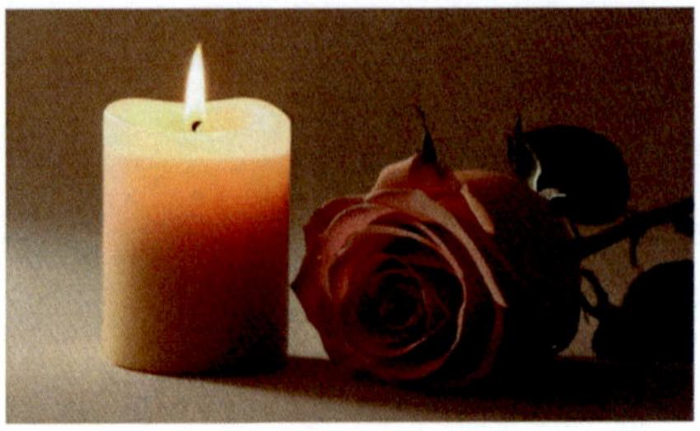

When we think of grief, we usually think of losing a loved one. But navigating a medical diagnosis brings its own deep, complex grief. You are mourning the loss of your "healthy identity," your independence, and your sense of control. Failing to recognize and name this as grief can leave you feeling stuck and overwhelmed.

Here are practical, research-backed ways to process this season:

- **Name It to Tame It:** Simply saying, "I am grieving the loss of my normal life right now," shifts your brain out of the fight-or-flight response and allows you to process the emotion.
- **Acknowledge Anticipatory Grief:** Grief expert David Kessler explains "anticipatory grief"—when our minds jump to the future to imagine the worst-case scenario. When this panic hits, gently bring your focus back to today. Say to yourself, "In this exact moment, we are safe."
- **Start a Grief Journal:** Write down exactly what you feel you have lost. Later, as you process and heal, go back to those pages and write down what you have gained (new strength, perspective, or deeper relationships).
- **Prioritize Physical Rest:** Grief isn't just an emotional weight; it is a physical one. Processing trauma and loss is exhausting for your body. Give yourself permission to sleep more, rest often, and lower your daily expectations. Exhaustion is a natural symptom of grief, not a sign of weakness.
- **Hold Space for Both:** You can hold space for grief while still moving forward. Use the Wins & Milestones and Glimmers of Gratitude trackers at the back of this book to celebrate your daily progress. Acknowledge the loss and celebrate the steps forward.
- **Seek Low-Pressure Support:** Don't wait until remission to get help. Talk to your hospital's oncology social worker, or schedule a teletherapy session (we did this via Zoom right from the hospital room). If you try an in-person or virtual support group, remove the pressure: you can always attend one session and leave if it isn't the right fit for you.

### A Note from Lindsey:

Grief isn't just for the patient. As a care partner, your entire world has been upended, too. You are grieving the loss of your routine, the shift in your relationship, and your peace of mind. Please know that your grief is 100% valid. I maintained my own separate counseling appointments during Thomas' treatment, and I cannot stress this enough: seeking support is not a luxury; it is a necessity. It is the classic airplane rule: you have to put your own oxygen mask on first before assisting anyone else. Please take care of your heart, too.

# Cultivating Gratitude

Research shows gratitude is a powerful tool for building emotional resilience, reducing stress, and finding peace. However, being told to "just look on the bright side" can feel dismissive. Genuine gratitude doesn't mean ignoring the hard things; it means actively looking for good things, too. In our own journey, we incorporated gratitude into our prayer time, thanking God for the blessings in the midst of challenges.

**Ways to Foster Gratitude:**

- **"Three Good Things":** Writing down three positive things daily can rewire your brain to scan for the good. Use the *Moments of Gratitude* log at the back of this book to start.

- **Thank Your Care Team:** Say thank you, write a card, or nominate a caregiver for a hospital award—like a DAISY Award for exceptional nurses or a ROSE Award for amazing support staff (ask your hospital staff how to submit a nomination). Look back at your *Care Team Connections* pages and check off the names of those you thank or nominate. Keeping a dish of chocolates by your hospital door or bringing treats to the staff station are also great ways to express gratitude!

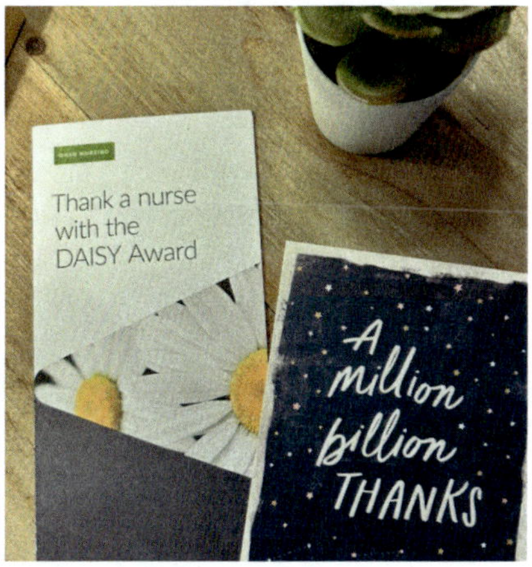


- **Find "Pockets of Joy":** You don't need a grand vacation to experience joy. When you are keenly aware of how precious life is, ordinary moments take on an extraordinary beauty. Seek out these small delights, like watching a favorite movie, eating a special meal, or simply sitting outside to feel the breeze.

- **Say What Matters Most:** Don't wait for the perfect moment—make a call, send a text, say "I love you," or extend forgiveness today. You can also look through your phone at happy memories and send a favorite photo to someone who shared the experience with you.

### A Note from Thomas

When my mom, Julie, received a terminal diagnosis, she became my model for navigating adversity with joy. In fact, one of her very first questions for her oncologist was, "Can we go to Disneyland before treatment starts?"

We cherished those magical days on vacation, but she also taught me you don't need a theme park to find happiness. She proved that no matter your prognosis, you still hold the power to choose how you want to live today. After she passed, we dedicated a bench in her honor at her favorite spot in Bend, Drake Park. The plaque reads: "Live Fully, Laugh Often, Love Always."

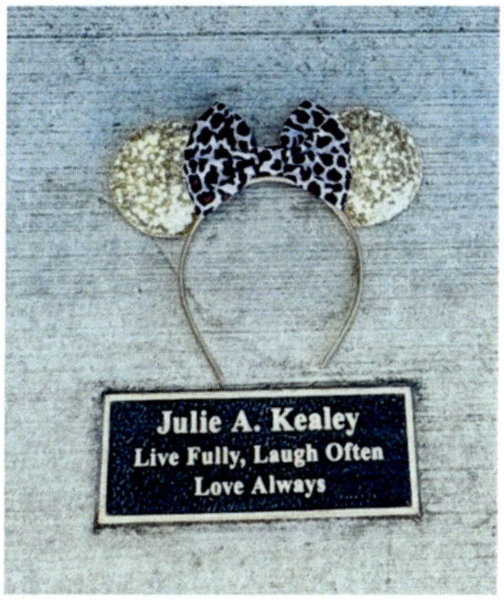

# HOPE-FILLED *Phrases*

## Do the next right thing.

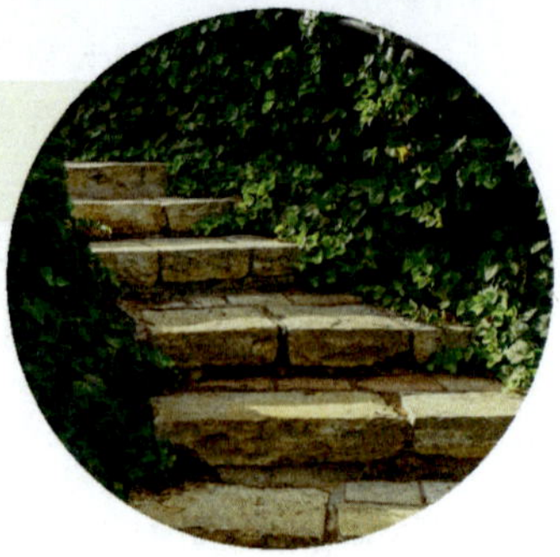

When facing an overwhelming big picture, break down your challenges into manageable steps, helping you find clarity and control.

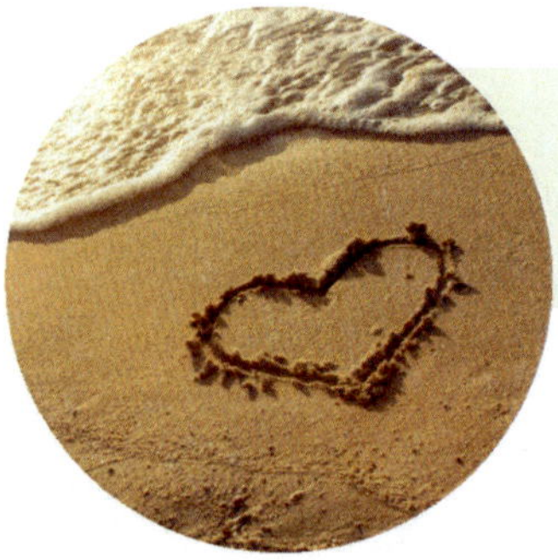

## Treat yourself as you would treat a good friend.

When you are having a hard time, give yourself the same grace and kindness you would offer a loved one.

## I can do hard things.

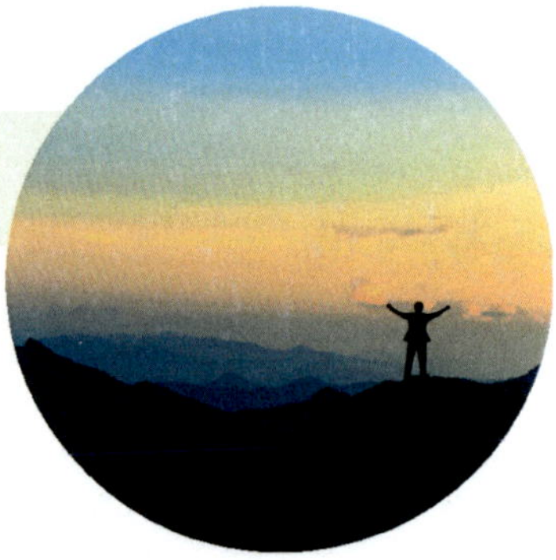

This shifts your brain from a state of fear to a state of agency, reminding you that you have already survived 100% of your hardest days.

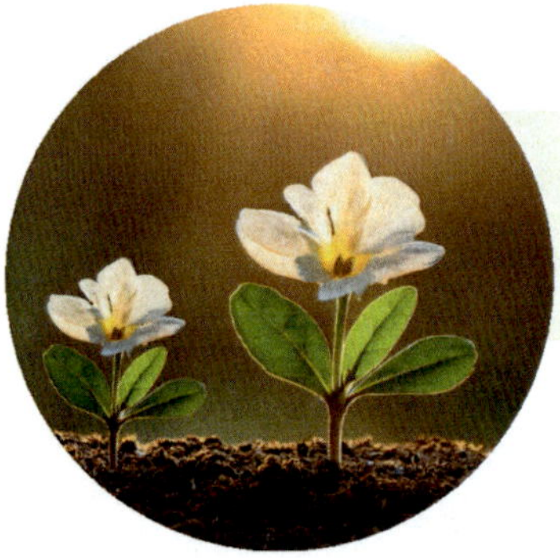

## If I'm going to go through this, I want to grow through this.

This empowers you to be an active participant in your journey, allowing you to find purpose in your pain.

## I am not alone.

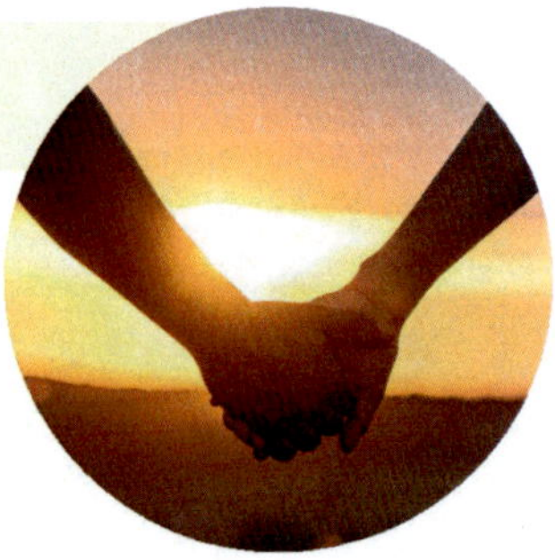

Even in your hardest moments, you are being carried by a greater community, be it through family, friendship, or faith.

# MY ANCHORS OF *Encouragement*

Use the space below to write the quotes, thoughts, or phrases that encourage you and bring you hope. Scan the QR code on page 5 to see the Bible verses that brought Thomas and Lindsey comfort throughout their health journey.

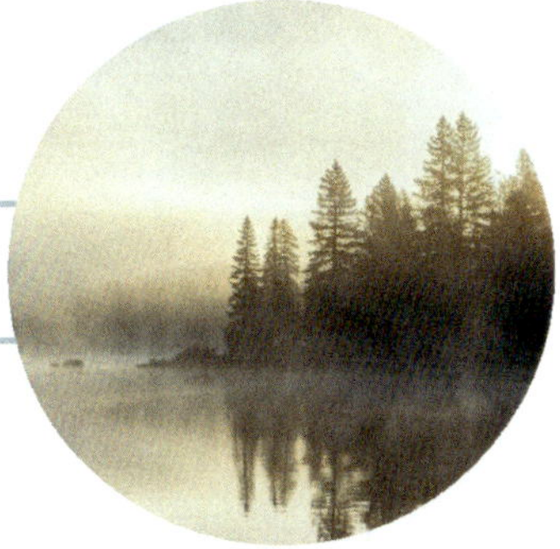

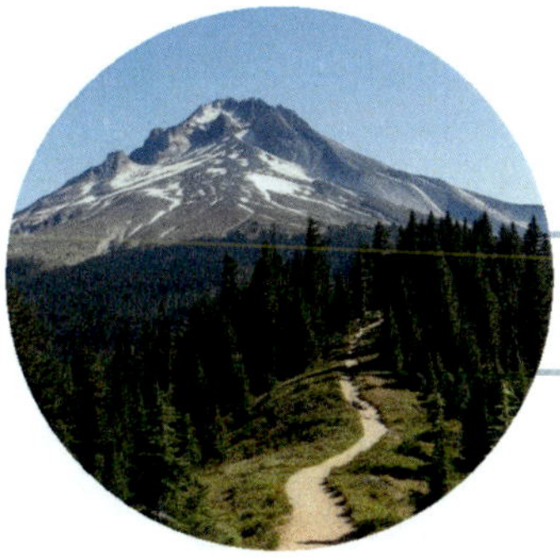

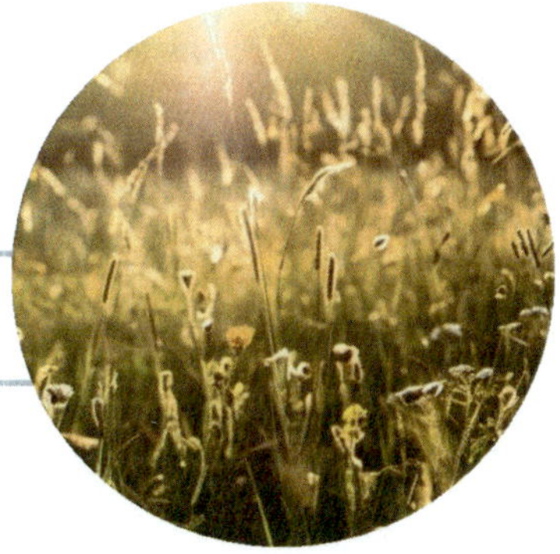

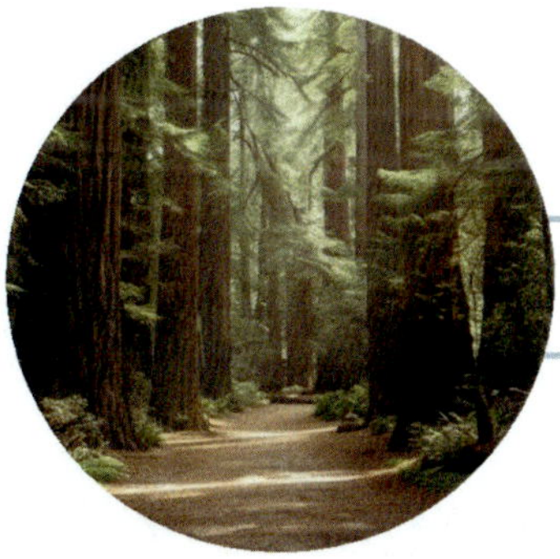

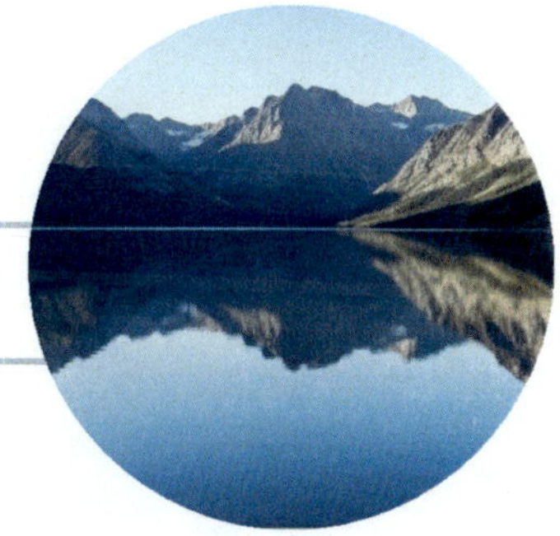

# GIVE YOURSELF GRACE.

# PART 4

# THE ROAD HOME

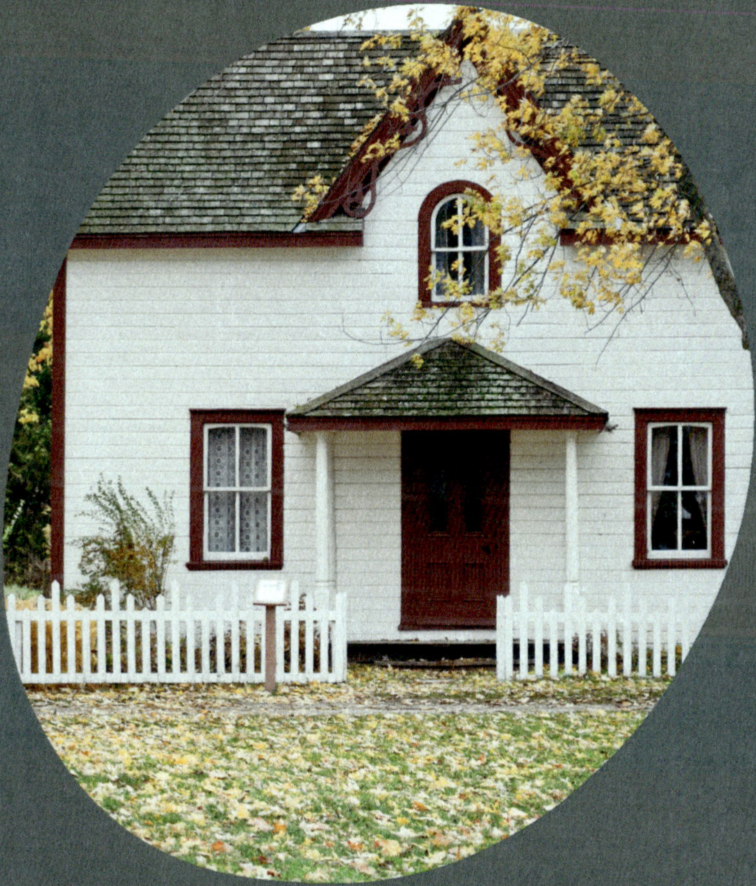

## Promoting Health Beyond the Hospital

# Navigating the Transition from Hospital to Home

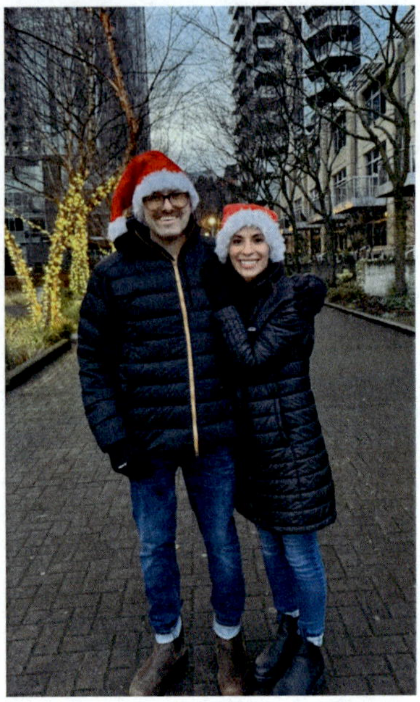

Walking out of the hospital doors is the goal, but it brings a new challenge. You are leaving a controlled environment where you were monitored 24/7 and entering a world where you and your Care Partner are the captains. Recovery doesn't end when you leave the unit. In fact, the work you do at home—how you eat, how you move, and how you set up your space—is what rebuilds your body.

**Give Yourself Grace**

Going "solo" is a massive adjustment. You are suddenly taking on the roles of pharmacist, nurse, and scheduler without a call button to push. You will not be perfect on Day 1. If you fumble a medication time or feel overwhelmed by the silence of the house, take a breath. You are learning a brand new way of living, and it is okay to be a beginner.

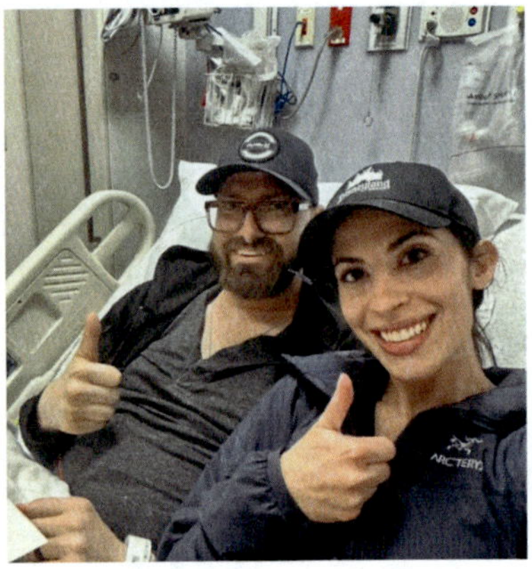

**When in Doubt, Reach Out**

Use the Patient Portal (MyChart) for non-urgent questions, but for fevers or concerning changes, call the clinic immediately (you should have a list of symptoms to call about). Unplanned returns to the ER for neutropenic fevers are often part of the process, so do not panic. Thomas had many ER admissions (even on New Year's Eve), and we made it through every single one.

***Pro-Tip:*** *If you are heading to the ER, call your clinic first. Ask them to alert the ER that you are immunocompromised so you can bypass the general waiting room and go straight to a "safe" area away from other sick patients.*

**What's In This Section:**

- **Eating the Rainbow:** A guide to help you visualize how different colors of food support your healing (consult your doctor or dietitian before making any dietary changes)
- **Socializing Safely:** Creative hacks for connecting with loved ones while staying protected and immunocompromised
- **Movement & Grace:** Gentle, baby-step strategies to help you rebuild your physical strength and combat "chemo brain" at your own pace
- **Home & Recovery List:** A curated list of the items we used for recovery
- **Habit Tracker:** A sample tracker to show you how small, daily choices compound into massive healing over time

# Socializing Safely While Immunocompromised

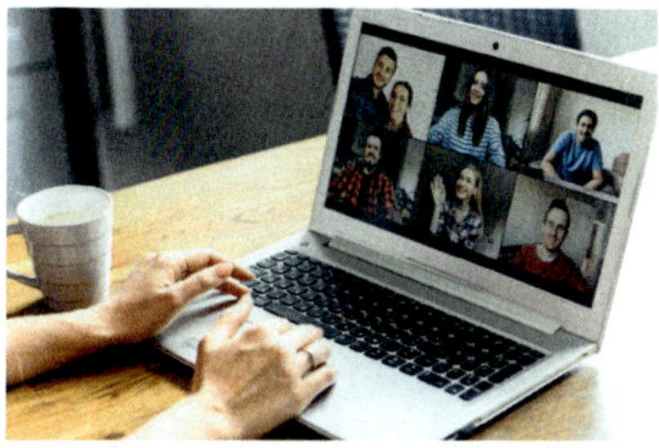

Research shows that social connection is vital to your overall healing, mental health, and even your immune system. Prolonged isolation can take a heavy toll on your body, which means completely cutting yourself off isn't the answer—you just have to get creative! Always consult your doctor for specific health and safety guidelines regarding your immune system and safe socializing.

**1. Establish Your "Social Parameters"**

Friends and loved ones often assume that once you are discharged, life can simply "go back to normal." But your blood counts might fluctuate during recovery, and those numbers may dictate how you can safely interact. Take the pressure off yourself by "blaming" your medical team. We would tell friends: "Thomas' current socializing parameters are..." explaining that our plans were strictly based on his doctor's recommendations. (E.g., For now, Thomas cannot do in-person indoor visits for the time being, guests must wear masks, anyone with a sniffle, cough, or recent sick contacts cannot visit, etc.).

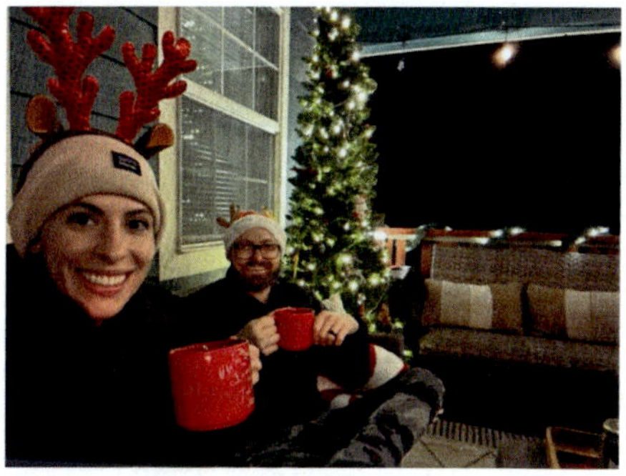

**2. Create a Safe Gathering Space**

Outdoor gatherings can be much safer. Living in the Pacific Northwest, we converted our front porch into a socially distanced hangout. We hosted small "Polar Porch Parties" with battery-powered heated seats, blankets, space heaters, and warm drinks to see friends without sharing indoor air!

**3. The Host's Toolkit**

Make it easy for guests to follow the rules by keeping these by the front door:

- **Colorful Masks:** We provided multicolored N95s/KN95s. It meant guests didn't have to bring their own, and the colors made masking feel less clinical.
- **Hospital-Grade Sanitizer:** We bought on Amazon big pump bottles of moisturizing 3M hand sanitizer (what the hospitals use) for guests to use upon arrival.
- **At-Home Tests:** When his blood counts were low, we gave COVID/Flu A/B tests as stocking stuffers! We asked family to test before seeing us to catch asymptomatic carriers.

**4. Holiday Hacks & Virtual Fun**

You don't have to cancel the holidays; just get creative!

- **Themed Zooms:** Host virtual family gatherings where everyone wears Santa hats or birthday crowns.
- **Halloween Safety:** Immunocompromised patients shouldn't carve real pumpkins (due to mold/bacteria risks), so we carved fake ones from Target! On Halloween we also set a candy table on the sidewalk and waved to trick-or-treaters from the porch.

# Movement & Grace: Befriending Your Body

Before cancer, Thomas was a hiker, mountain biker, and weight lifter. But post-transplant, he had lost 40 pounds. Severe anemia meant his blood wasn't fully oxygenated, leading to dizziness and impacted stability. We had to learn a massive lesson in extending grace to ourselves.

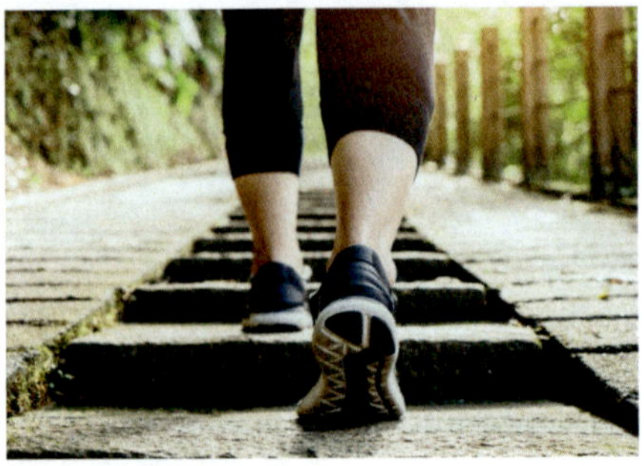

If you are in this season, please know that your fitness level will look different right now, and that is completely okay. Here are some practical ways to approach movement during recovery. Always consult your doctor before starting any exercise routine.

**1. Embrace the "Baby Steps"**

- **Get the Gear:** We ordered a cane off Amazon for the days after discharge, and it was a game-changer for his stability. Celebrate the small progress—even if it's just walking to the mailbox!
- **Honor Your Hardware:** Thomas had a PICC line for quite a while due to frequent blood transfusions, meaning he couldn't lift anything over 10 pounds. Listen to your body and respect your medical restrictions. It is an amazing feeling when those lines finally come out!
- **Ask for a PT Referral:** Ask your doctor for a referral to a Physical Therapist, ideally one with experience working with oncology patients. A good PT will understand that healing isn't linear and will help you safely rebuild your strength at your own pace.

**2. The "Counterintuitive" Energy Boost**

When you are exhausted from treatment, taking a walk usually does not sound fun. But counterintuitively, if it is medically safe, movement can actually increase your energy!

- **The 5-Minute Rule:** Start with just a 5-minute walk.
- **The Post-Dinner Stroll:** A short walk after dinner actually helps your muscles metabolize sugar, preventing glucose spikes and energy crashes.

**3. Fighting "Chemo Brain"**

Treatments like chemotherapy and radiation can cause cognitive fog and memory issues. Physical exercise is actually one of the best ways to combat this!

- **Boost Your BDNF:** Exercise triggers the release of BDNF (Brain-Derived Neurotrophic Factor), a protein that helps to repair and grow new neural connections.
- **Cross-Train Your Mind:** Combine physical movement with cognitive exercises. Doing brain games, reading, or practicing a new language are excellent ways to keep your brain sharp while your body heals.

# Nourishing Your Body

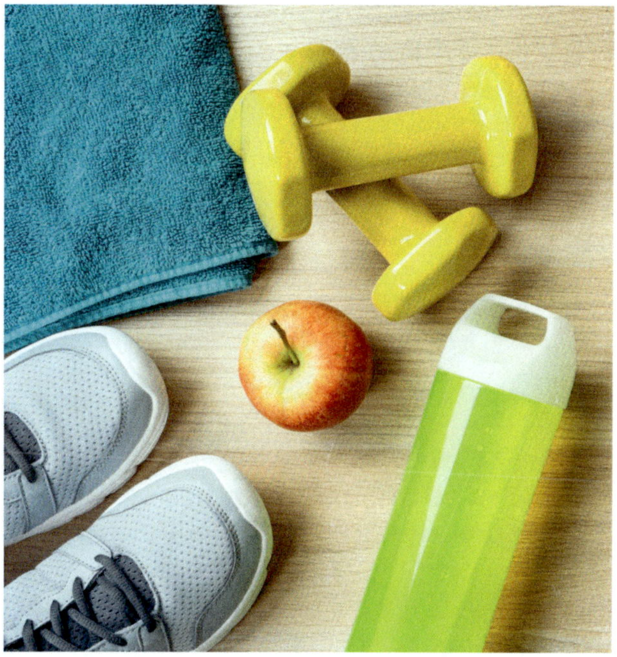

When you're facing intense medical treatments like chemotherapy, proper nutrition and hydration become absolutely vital for healing, but they can also be incredibly challenging. Appetite can disappear, nausea can strike, and fatigue can make even the simplest meal prep feel impossible. That's why we put together this list of items, specifically designed to make it easier to nourish your body, stay hydrated, and incorporate gentle movement, even on your lowest energy days after discharging from the hospital.

When we were living at the Ronald McDonald House in a small studio apartment post-transplant, every item on this list earned its spot because it fit in our limited space and we used it daily.

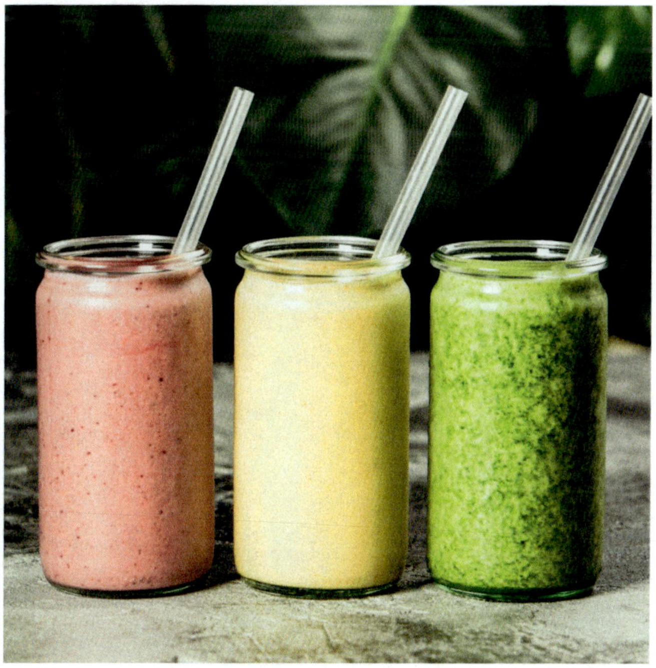

Dietary restrictions are also a big part of the post-transplant journey. For us, smoothies were, and continue to be, the name of the game! Initially, Thomas couldn't have things like spinach or yogurt, but we still packed them with frozen berries, bananas, and other safe ingredients, gradually expanding as his diet allowed. They're also fantastic for adding protein powder. And since he couldn't eat raw vegetables for the first 100 days, our Ninja Air Fryer was an absolute lifesaver, allowing us to easily cook vegetables safely. To give you inspiration to eat healthy and diverse foods, we even created "The Power of Eating the Rainbow" page, which we printed and put on our refrigerator.

# THE POWER OF *Eating the Rainbow*

**Consult with your doctor or registered dietitian before making any dietary changes. If you are immunocompromised, ask your care team about their specific guidelines for consuming fresh produce, as neutropenic diet protocols can vary.*

## Red

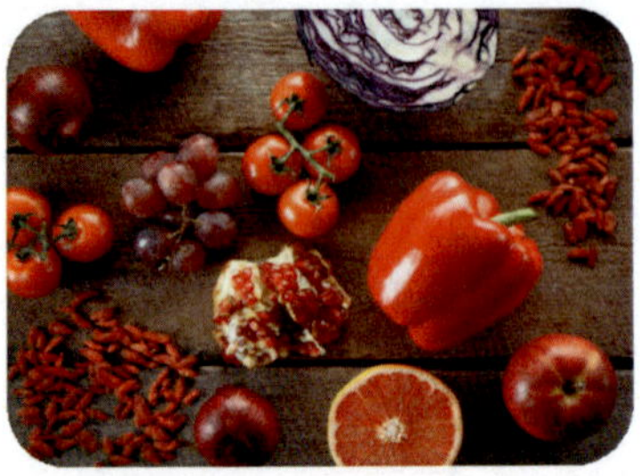

Rich in lycopene and anthocyanins, red fruits and veggies are fantastic for heart health, offering support for blood pressure and cholesterol. They're also powerful antioxidants. Examples: Tomatoes, Strawberries, Red Bell Peppers, Beets.

## Orange

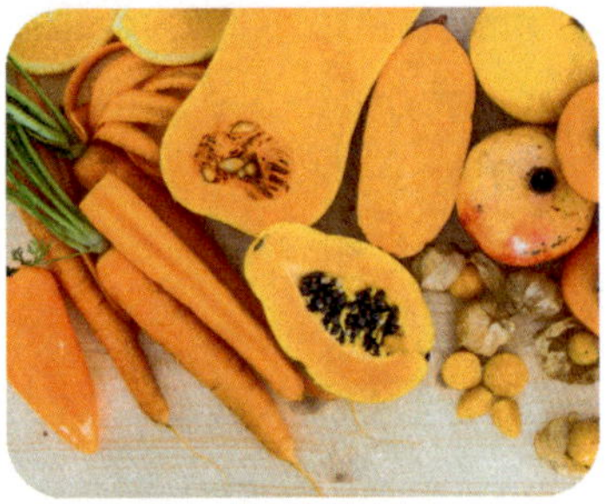

Packed with carotenoids like beta-carotene, orange produce gives a major boost to your immune system and promotes vibrant skin health. They are also key for good vision and have anti-inflammatory properties. Examples: Carrots, Sweet Potatoes, Oranges, Mangoes, Pumpkin.

## Yellow

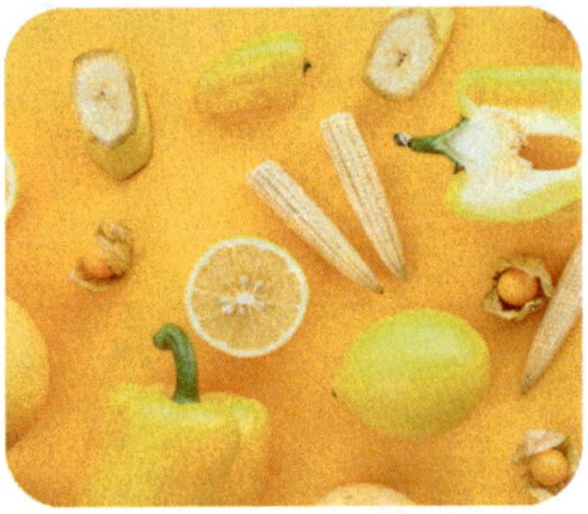

High in Vitamin C, lutein, and zeaxanthin, yellow fruits and veggies are essential for strong immune function and excellent eye health. They help protect cells and support overall vitality. Examples: Lemons, Pineapple, Yellow Bell Peppers, Corn, Bananas.

## Green

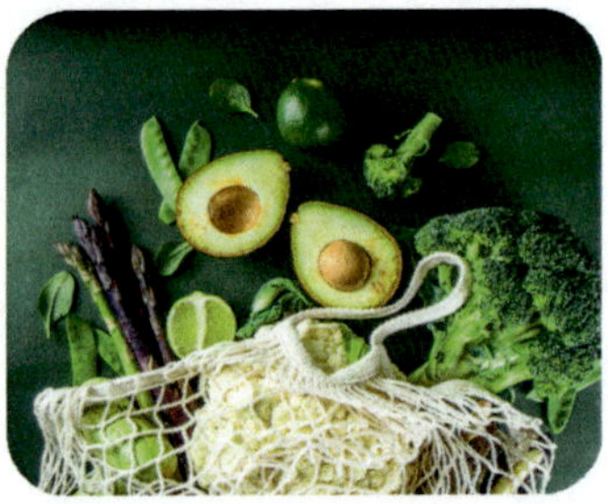

Thanks to chlorophyll, folate, and Vitamin K, green fruits and veggies are excellent for detoxification support, strong bones, and healthy digestion. They also provide strong immune and cellular protection. Examples: Spinach, Kale, Broccoli, Asparagus, Avocado.

## Blue & Purple

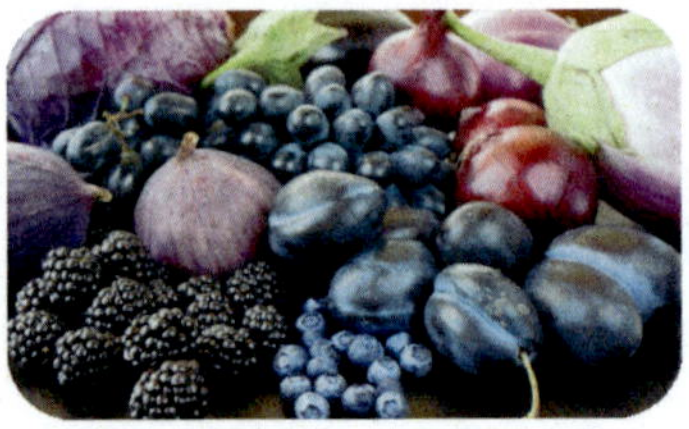

High in anthocyanins and resveratrol, these foods are champions for brain power, memory, and overall anti-aging effects. Examples: Blueberries, Blackberries, Grapes, Eggplant, Purple Cabbage.

# Habit Tracker

| Week of: | Monday | Tuesday | Wednesday | Thursday | Friday | Saturday | Sunday |
|---|---|---|---|---|---|---|---|

HEALTHY FOOD

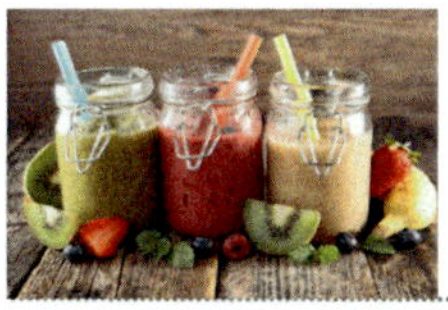

WALK/EXERCISE

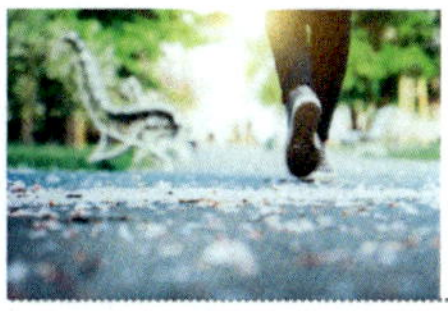

STRETCH

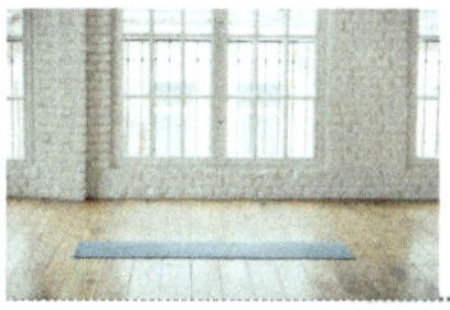

QUALITY SLEEP

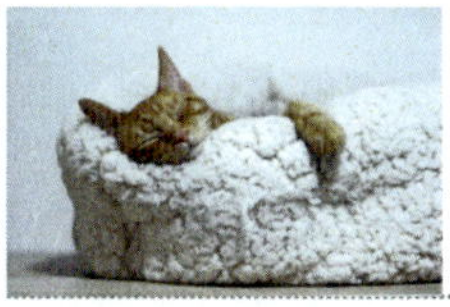

READ/BRAIN CHALLENGE

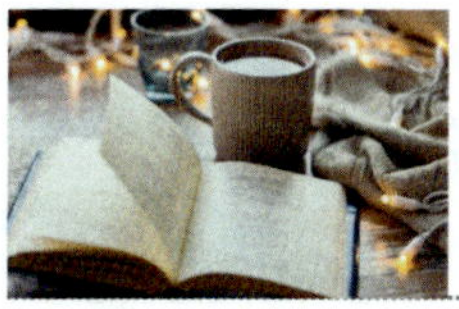

OTHER:

# Home & Recovery List

## Clothing & Protection

- ○ PICC Access Sweatshirt
- ○ Waterproof PICC Sleeve
- ○ Wide Brim Sun Hat
- ○ UV Shirt: Critical sun protection if you are navigating GVHD or photosensitivity
- ○ KN95/N95 Face Masks
- ○ Compression Socks

## Mouth & Eye Care

- ○ Wisdom Teeth Syringe: Essential for gently rinsing food out of mouth sores (from chemo) without touching them.
- ○ Biotene Spray / XyliMelts: A lifesaver for "Dry Mouth" to help you sleep.
- ○ Preservative-Free Eye Drops

## Nutrition & Diet

- ○ Air Fryer: Perfect for cooking vegetables to a safe temperature without a full kitchen (raw veggies may not be allowed while neutropenic or during the first 100+ days post-transplant)
- ○ Blender: For high-protein smoothies when chewing is hard.

## Comfort for Symptoms

- ○ Neck fan & Ice Beanie (for chemo hot flashes)
- ○ Peppermint Essential Oil Roller (for Nausea)
- ○ Chemo Headwear
- ○ Wisdom Teeth Ice Pack Wrap (for mucositis)
- ○ Cooling Comfort Blanket

## Air & Water Safety

- ○ Air Purifier: A medical-grade filter to remove mold and viruses from your recovery room. (We use AirDoctor).
- ○ Water Purifier: Countertop reverse-osmosis system to ensure your water is free of contaminants.

## Strength & Movement

- ○ Neoprene Hand Weights
- ○ Under-Desk Treadmill
- ○ Walking Cane: Helpful for stability as you regain strength.

Product Links

# Recommended Wellness Items

Rebuilding your physical health is a slow, steady process that requires the right tools for your environment. These resources were instrumental in helping us manage nutrition and stay active during the most challenging phases of treatment.

Product Links

**Please Note:** Always consult your hospital's registered dietitian or your transplant team before introducing new foods or using outside cooking appliances (like air fryers or blenders) to ensure they meet your current safety and sterilization requirements.

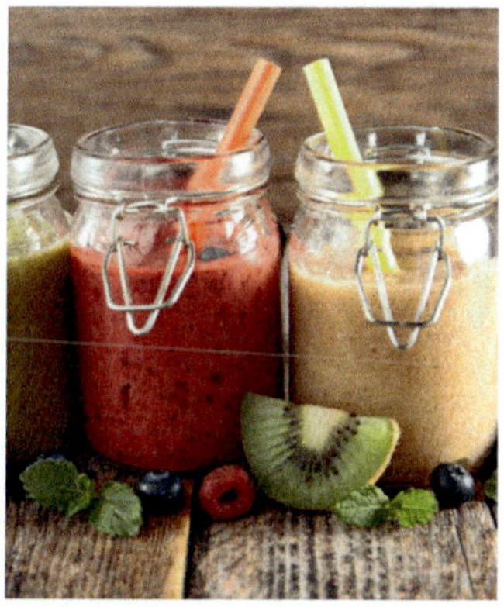

- **Blender**: Great for easy smoothies, protein shakes, or blending soft foods when appetite is low or chewing is difficult.
- **Countertop Water Purifier**: Ensure you have access to clean, great-tasting water (we use Aqua TRU Carafe).
- **Air Purifier**: Provides medical-grade air filtration to capture ultra-fine particles, allergens, mold spores, bacteria, and viruses, creating a cleaner and safer breathing environment, especially important for immunocompromised patients (we use AirDoctor).
- **Air Fry Countertop Oven**: Perfect for safely cooking vegetables and other foods in small spaces, especially when dietary restrictions prevent eating raw options (we use Ninja).
- **Water Bottle Carrier Holder**: Staying hydrated is key; having a favorite bottle and carrier helps.
- **Neoprene Dumbbell Hand Weights**: Light exercise and staying active can be beneficial for strength and mood, even in limited spaces.
- **Under Desk Treadmill**: A compact and portable option for gentle walking and movement, even in small hospital or temporary living spaces, to help maintain strength.

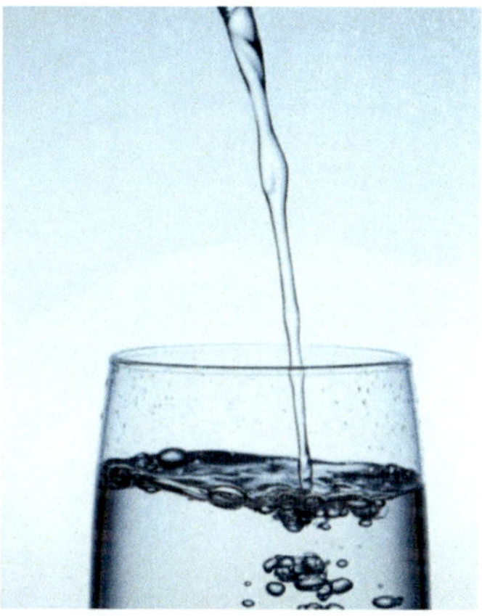

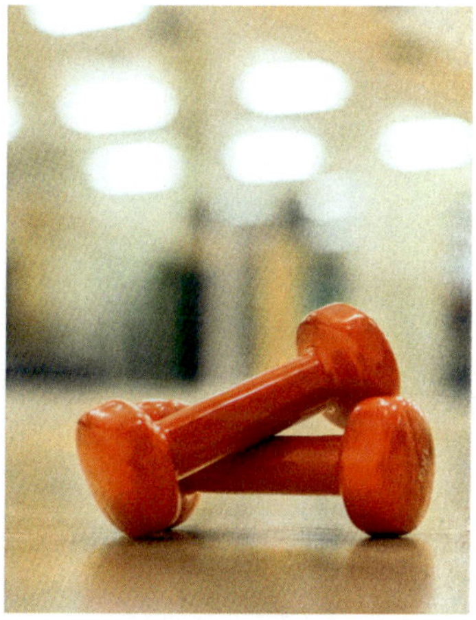

# CELEBRATE EVERY VICTORY.

PART 5

# The Daily Navigator

Templates and Trackers

# Your Logbook for Progress and Gratitude

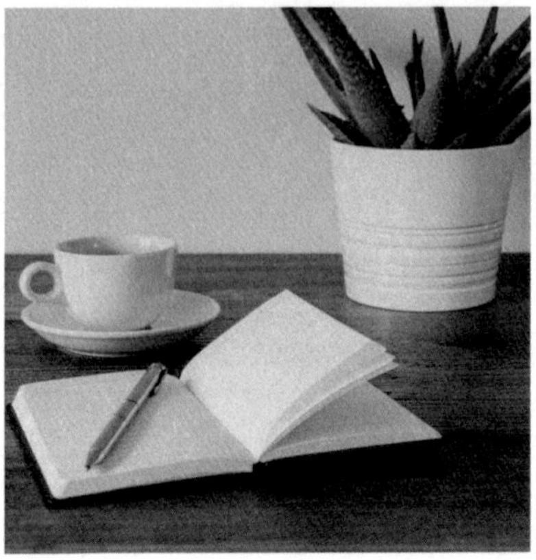

## How to Use This Section

Recovery is not a straight line. Some days you will have the energy to track every vital sign; other days, you might only have the energy to write down one good thing that happened. That is okay. We designed this section to be modular, meaning you can use the pages that serve you best in the moment. Use what helps, leave what doesn't, and trust your own rhythm.

If you run out of tracker pages and want to keep your journal going, scan the QR code to download and print free copies of these templates.

## Your Navigator Tools:

- **Wins & Milestones:** This running log is a place to capture wins—whether it was "walked two laps," "ate a popsicle," or "got discharged." Seeing these lines stack up over time provides powerful visual proof of your resilience.
- **Moments of Gratitude:** Training your brain to find the light in the dark is a critical part of healing. There are no rules: write down one specific moment, list three things you are thankful for, or fill a whole page when you are feeling reflective.
- **Treatment & Milestone Calendar (12 Months):** A big-picture, monthly view to track treatment cycles, scan dates, and monthly goals throughout the year.
- **The Daily Health Tracker (30 Days):** Use these pages to log your labs, symptoms, and questions during acute, intensive phases of treatment (like a hospital stay). On low-energy days, give yourself permission to skip the data and focus entirely on rest.
- **Weekly Health Log (12 Weeks):** Designed for the "step-down" phase of your journey. Whether you are transitioning home after a hospital stay or simply managing an ongoing outpatient routine, use these pages to log weekly trends, appointments, and the day-to-day adjustments of healing.

# Wins & Milestones

Don't wait for the finish line to celebrate. In this journey, every small step forward is a massive victory. (Examples: Walked 2 laps around unit! Ate 1st solid food since TPN. PICC Line Out! Clear bone marrow biopsy!)

| DATE | THE WIN |
| --- | --- |
| | |
| | |
| | |
| | |
| | |
| | |
| | |
| | |
| | |
| | |
| | |
| | |
| | |
| | |
| | |

# Wins & Milestones

In treatment, there are no small victories. Every lap, every bite, and every stable lab report is a mountain climbed.

**DATE** **THE WIN**

# Wins & Milestones

Progress isn't always a straight line, but every forward step counts. Track the triumphs and honor the effort.

**DATE** **THE WIN**

# Wins & Milestones

Victory isn't just the finish line; it's every hard step you take to get there. Celebrate the progress, no matter the pace.

**DATE** **THE WIN**

# Wins & Milestones

Some days the win is a mile; some days the win is an inch. Both get you closer to the finish line. Track the triumphs and honor the effort it took to get there.

**DATE** **THE WIN**

# Wins & Milestones

These milestones are the evidence of your strength. Look back often to see how far you've actually come.

| DATE | THE WIN |
| --- | --- |
| | |
| | |
| | |
| | |
| | |
| | |
| | |
| | |
| | |
| | |
| | |
| | |
| | |
| | |
| | |

# Wins & Milestones

Focus on the step you are taking, not the distance left to go. Progress is progress, no matter how small. Record the effort and trust the process.

| DATE | THE WIN |
| --- | --- |
| | |
| | |
| | |
| | |
| | |
| | |
| | |
| | |
| | |
| | |
| | |
| | |
| | |
| | |
| | |

# *Moments of Gratitude*

Look for the glimmers—those tiny moments of connection and joy.
(Examples: A warm blanket fresh from the warmer. The first sip of coffee. Good laugh with the night nurse. A beautiful view out the window.)

| DATE | GRATITUDES |
| --- | --- |
| | |
| | |
| | |
| | |
| | |
| | |
| | |
| | |
| | |
| | |
| | |
| | |
| | |
| | |
| | |

# *Moments of Gratitude*

Glimmers aren't about pretending things are perfect; they're about finding the light that's already there.

**DATE** **GRATITUDES**

# Moments of Gratitude

Gratitude isn't about ignoring the pain; it's about finding the beauty that exists alongside it. Even on the hardest days, look for the light.

| DATE | GRATITUDES |
| --- | --- |
| | |
| | |
| | |
| | |
| | |
| | |
| | |
| | |
| | |
| | |
| | |
| | |
| | |
| | |
| | |

# Moments of Gratitude

"It's not joy that makes us grateful. It's gratitude that makes us joyful." — Brené Brown

**DATE** **GRATITUDES**

# Moments of Gratitude

Gratitude doesn't change the circumstances, but it changes the person standing in the middle of them.

**DATE** **GRATITUDES**

# *Moments of Gratitude*

In a sea of "what ifs," gratitude is the "what is." Find one small thing that is true, good, and right here with you in this moment.

**DATE** **GRATITUDES**

# Moments of Gratitude

A gratitude doesn't have to be big to be meaningful. A cold drink, a soft blanket, or a text from home—if it brought you a second of peace, it belongs here.

**DATE** **GRATITUDES**

# Treatment & Milestone Calendar

Month: ____________________

| SUNDAY | MONDAY | TUESDAY | WEDNESDAY | THURSDAY | FRIDAY | SATURDAY |
|---|---|---|---|---|---|---|
| | | | | | | |
| | | | | | | |
| | | | | | | |
| | | | | | | |
| | | | | | | |
| | | | | | | |

MONTHLY GOALS

# Treatment & Milestone Calendar

Month: ____________________________

| SUNDAY | MONDAY | TUESDAY | WEDNESDAY | THURSDAY | FRIDAY | SATURDAY |
|---|---|---|---|---|---|---|
| | | | | | | |
| | | | | | | |
| | | | | | | |
| | | | | | | |
| | | | | | | |
| | | | | | | |

**MONTHLY GOALS**

# Treatment & Milestone Calendar

Month: ______________________

| SUNDAY | MONDAY | TUESDAY | WEDNESDAY | THURSDAY | FRIDAY | SATURDAY |
|---|---|---|---|---|---|---|
| | | | | | | |
| | | | | | | |
| | | | | | | |
| | | | | | | |
| | | | | | | |
| | | | | | | |

MONTHLY GOALS

# Treatment & Milestone Calendar

Month: ______________________

| SUNDAY | MONDAY | TUESDAY | WEDNESDAY | THURSDAY | FRIDAY | SATURDAY |
|---|---|---|---|---|---|---|
| | | | | | | |
| | | | | | | |
| | | | | | | |
| | | | | | | |
| | | | | | | |
| | | | | | | |

MONTHLY GOALS

# Treatment & Milestone Calendar

Month: ______________________

| SUNDAY | MONDAY | TUESDAY | WEDNESDAY | THURSDAY | FRIDAY | SATURDAY |
| --- | --- | --- | --- | --- | --- | --- |
| | | | | | | |
| | | | | | | |
| | | | | | | |
| | | | | | | |
| | | | | | | |
| | | | | | | |

MONTHLY GOALS

# Treatment & Milestone Calendar

Month: ____________________

| SUNDAY | MONDAY | TUESDAY | WEDNESDAY | THURSDAY | FRIDAY | SATURDAY |
|---|---|---|---|---|---|---|
| | | | | | | |
| | | | | | | |
| | | | | | | |
| | | | | | | |
| | | | | | | |
| | | | | | | |

MONTHLY GOALS

# Treatment & Milestone Calendar

Month: ______________________________

| SUNDAY | MONDAY | TUESDAY | WEDNESDAY | THURSDAY | FRIDAY | SATURDAY |
|---|---|---|---|---|---|---|
| | | | | | | |
| | | | | | | |
| | | | | | | |
| | | | | | | |
| | | | | | | |
| | | | | | | |

MONTHLY GOALS

# Treatment & Milestone Calendar

Month: ___________________________

| SUNDAY | MONDAY | TUESDAY | WEDNESDAY | THURSDAY | FRIDAY | SATURDAY |
|---|---|---|---|---|---|---|
| | | | | | | |
| | | | | | | |
| | | | | | | |
| | | | | | | |
| | | | | | | |
| | | | | | | |

MONTHLY GOALS

# Treatment & Milestone Calendar

Month: ____________________

| SUNDAY | MONDAY | TUESDAY | WEDNESDAY | THURSDAY | FRIDAY | SATURDAY |
|---|---|---|---|---|---|---|
| | | | | | | |
| | | | | | | |
| | | | | | | |
| | | | | | | |
| | | | | | | |
| | | | | | | |

MONTHLY GOALS

# Treatment & Milestone Calendar

*Month:* ______________________

| SUNDAY | MONDAY | TUESDAY | WEDNESDAY | THURSDAY | FRIDAY | SATURDAY |
|---|---|---|---|---|---|---|
| | | | | | | |
| | | | | | | |
| | | | | | | |
| | | | | | | |
| | | | | | | |
| | | | | | | |

**MONTHLY GOALS**

# Treatment & Milestone Calendar

Month: ______________________

| SUNDAY | MONDAY | TUESDAY | WEDNESDAY | THURSDAY | FRIDAY | SATURDAY |
|---|---|---|---|---|---|---|
| | | | | | | |
| | | | | | | |
| | | | | | | |
| | | | | | | |
| | | | | | | |
| | | | | | | |

MONTHLY GOALS

# Treatment & Milestone Calendar

Month: ____________________

| SUNDAY | MONDAY | TUESDAY | WEDNESDAY | THURSDAY | FRIDAY | SATURDAY |
|---|---|---|---|---|---|---|
| | | | | | | |
| | | | | | | |
| | | | | | | |
| | | | | | | |
| | | | | | | |
| | | | | | | |

MONTHLY GOALS

# Health Tracker

Date: ________ Day: Su M Tu W Th F Sa

**LABS & VITALS**

WBC: ______ Hemoglobin: ________ Platelets: ________ ANC: __________

Other: _____________ Other: ____________ Other: ______________

Temp: __________ Weight: __________ Other Vitals: ___________________

**SYMPTOMS**

Pain (0-10): ____ Fatigue (0-10): ____ Nausea (0-10): ____

Other (Rash, GI, Mouth Sores, etc.): ________________________________

**DAILY LIVING**

Sleep: ____ hrs Water: ______ oz BM: ______

Movement: ____________________________________________________

Appetite / Meals: _______________________________________________

Today's Treatment: ______________________________________________

Today's Small Win: ______________________________________________

**CARE TEAM & NOTES**

Nurse(s): _________________ Provider(s): _________________

Questions/Notes:

# Health Tracker

Date: ________ Day: Su M Tu W Th F Sa

## LABS & VITALS

WBC: ______ Hemoglobin: ________ Platelets: ________ ANC: __________

Other: ____________ Other: ____________ Other: ____________

Temp: __________ Weight: __________ Other Vitals: ____________________

## SYMPTOMS

Pain (0-10): ____ Fatigue (0-10): ____ Nausea (0-10): ____

Other (Rash, GI, Mouth Sores, etc.): ______________________________

## DAILY LIVING

Sleep: ____ hrs Water: ______ oz BM: ______

Movement: ____________________________________________

Appetite / Meals: ______________________________________

Today's Treatment: _____________________________________

Today's Small Win: _____________________________________

## CARE TEAM & NOTES

Nurse(s): ________________ Provider(s): ________________

Questions/Notes:

# Health Tracker

Date: ________ Day: Su M Tu W Th F Sa

## LABS & VITALS

WBC: ______ Hemoglobin: ________ Platelets: ________ ANC: __________

Other: ______________ Other: _____________ Other: _______________

Temp: __________ Weight: __________ Other Vitals: ____________________

## SYMPTOMS

Pain (0-10): ____ Fatigue (0-10): ____ Nausea (0-10): ____

Other (Rash, GI, Mouth Sores, etc.): ____________________________________

## DAILY LIVING

Sleep: ____ hrs Water: ______ oz BM: ______

Movement: ____________________________________________________

Appetite / Meals: ______________________________________________

Today's Treatment: ____________________________________________

Today's Small Win: ____________________________________________

## CARE TEAM & NOTES

Nurse(s): __________________ Provider(s): __________________

Questions/Notes:

____________________________________________________________

____________________________________________________________

____________________________________________________________

____________________________________________________________

____________________________________________________________

____________________________________________________________

____________________________________________________________

# Health Tracker

Date: ________ Day: Su M Tu W Th F Sa

**LABS & VITALS**

WBC: ______ Hemoglobin: ________ Platelets: ________ ANC: __________

Other: _____________ Other: ____________ Other: ______________

Temp: __________ Weight: __________ Other Vitals: ___________________

**SYMPTOMS**

Pain (0-10): ____ Fatigue (0-10): ____ Nausea (0-10): ____

Other (Rash, GI, Mouth Sores, etc.): ________________________________

**DAILY LIVING**

Sleep: ____ hrs Water: ______ oz BM: ______

Movement: ____________________________________________________

Appetite / Meals: _______________________________________________

Today's Treatment: ______________________________________________

Today's Small Win: ______________________________________________

**CARE TEAM & NOTES**

Nurse(s): _________________ Provider(s): _________________

Questions/Notes:

______________________________________________________________

______________________________________________________________

______________________________________________________________

______________________________________________________________

______________________________________________________________

______________________________________________________________

______________________________________________________________

# Health Tracker

Date: ________

Day: Su M Tu W Th F Sa

## LABS & VITALS

WBC: ______ Hemoglobin: ________ Platelets: ________ ANC: __________

Other: ______________ Other: _____________ Other: _______________

Temp: __________ Weight: __________ Other Vitals: ____________________

## SYMPTOMS

Pain (0-10): ____ Fatigue (0-10): ____ Nausea (0-10): ____

Other (Rash, GI, Mouth Sores, etc.): __________________________________

## DAILY LIVING

Sleep: ____ hrs Water: ______ oz BM: ______

Movement: _______________________________________________________

Appetite / Meals: ________________________________________________

Today's Treatment: _______________________________________________

Today's Small Win: _______________________________________________

## CARE TEAM & NOTES

Nurse(s): __________________ Provider(s): __________________

Questions/Notes:

_________________________________________________________________

_________________________________________________________________

_________________________________________________________________

_________________________________________________________________

_________________________________________________________________

_________________________________________________________________

_________________________________________________________________

# Health Tracker

Date: ________ Day: Su M Tu W Th F Sa

**LABS & VITALS**

WBC: ______ Hemoglobin: ________ Platelets: ________ ANC: __________

Other: ______________ Other: _____________ Other: _______________

Temp: __________ Weight: __________ Other Vitals: ____________________

**SYMPTOMS**

Pain (0-10): ____ Fatigue (0-10): ____ Nausea (0-10): ____

Other (Rash, GI, Mouth Sores, etc.): ________________________________

**DAILY LIVING**

Sleep: ____ hrs Water: ______ oz BM: ______

Movement: ______________________________________________________

Appetite / Meals: ________________________________________________

Today's Treatment: _______________________________________________

Today's Small Win: _______________________________________________

**CARE TEAM & NOTES**

Nurse(s): __________________ Provider(s): __________________

Questions/Notes:

_______________________________________________________________

_______________________________________________________________

_______________________________________________________________

_______________________________________________________________

_______________________________________________________________

_______________________________________________________________

_______________________________________________________________

# Health Tracker

Date: ________ Day: Su M Tu W Th F Sa

## LABS & VITALS

WBC: ______ Hemoglobin: ________ Platelets: ________ ANC: __________

Other: ______________ Other: _____________ Other: _______________

Temp: ___________ Weight: ___________ Other Vitals: ____________________

## SYMPTOMS

Pain (0-10): ____ Fatigue (0-10): ____ Nausea (0-10): ____

Other (Rash, GI, Mouth Sores, etc.): __________________________________

## DAILY LIVING

Sleep: ____ hrs Water: _______ oz BM: _______

Movement: ________________________________________________

Appetite / Meals: __________________________________________

Today's Treatment: _________________________________________

Today's Small Win: _________________________________________

## CARE TEAM & NOTES

Nurse(s): __________________ Provider(s): __________________

Questions/Notes:

_________________________________________________________________

_________________________________________________________________

_________________________________________________________________

_________________________________________________________________

_________________________________________________________________

_________________________________________________________________

_________________________________________________________________

# Health Tracker

Date: ________ Day: Su M Tu W Th F Sa

**LABS & VITALS**

WBC: ______ Hemoglobin: ________ Platelets: ________ ANC: __________

Other: _____________ Other: ____________ Other: ______________

Temp: __________ Weight: __________ Other Vitals: ___________________

**SYMPTOMS**

Pain (0-10): ____ Fatigue (0-10): ____ Nausea (0-10): ____

Other (Rash, GI, Mouth Sores, etc.): _________________________________

**DAILY LIVING**

Sleep: ____ hrs Water: ______ oz BM: ______

Movement: ______________________________________________________

Appetite / Meals: ________________________________________________

Today's Treatment: _______________________________________________

Today's Small Win: _______________________________________________

**CARE TEAM & NOTES**

Nurse(s): _________________ Provider(s): _________________

Questions/Notes:

# Health Tracker

Date: ________

Day: Su M Tu W Th F Sa

**LABS & VITALS**

WBC: ______ Hemoglobin: ________ Platelets: ________ ANC: __________

Other: _____________ Other: ____________ Other: ______________

Temp: __________ Weight: __________ Other Vitals: ___________________

**SYMPTOMS**

Pain (0-10): ____ Fatigue (0-10): ____ Nausea (0-10): ____

Other (Rash, GI, Mouth Sores, etc.): _________________________________

**DAILY LIVING**

Sleep: ____ hrs Water: ______ oz BM: ______

Movement: ______________________________________________________

Appetite / Meals: ________________________________________________

Today's Treatment: _______________________________________________

Today's Small Win: _______________________________________________

**CARE TEAM & NOTES**

Nurse(s): __________________ Provider(s): __________________

Questions/Notes:

_______________________________________________________________

_______________________________________________________________

_______________________________________________________________

_______________________________________________________________

_______________________________________________________________

_______________________________________________________________

_______________________________________________________________

# Health Tracker

Date: ________

Day: Su M Tu W Th F Sa

## LABS & VITALS

WBC: ______ Hemoglobin: ________ Platelets: ________ ANC: __________

Other: ______________ Other: ____________ Other: ______________

Temp: __________ Weight: __________ Other Vitals: ____________________

## SYMPTOMS

Pain (0-10): ____ Fatigue (0-10): ____ Nausea (0-10): ____

Other (Rash, GI, Mouth Sores, etc.): ________________________________

## DAILY LIVING

Sleep: ____ hrs Water: ______ oz BM: ______

Movement: ____________________________________________________

Appetite / Meals: _______________________________________________

Today's Treatment: ______________________________________________

Today's Small Win: ______________________________________________

## CARE TEAM & NOTES

Nurse(s): _________________ Provider(s): _________________

Questions/Notes:

____________________________________________________________

____________________________________________________________

____________________________________________________________

____________________________________________________________

____________________________________________________________

____________________________________________________________

____________________________________________________________

# Health Tracker

Date: ________ Day: Su M Tu W Th F Sa

## LABS & VITALS

WBC: ______ Hemoglobin: ________ Platelets: ________ ANC: __________

Other: ______________ Other: ____________ Other: ______________

Temp: __________ Weight: __________ Other Vitals: ___________________

## SYMPTOMS

Pain (0-10): ____ Fatigue (0-10): ____ Nausea (0-10): ____

Other (Rash, GI, Mouth Sores, etc.): ________________________________

## DAILY LIVING

Sleep: ____ hrs Water: ______ oz BM: ______

Movement: ______________________________________________________

Appetite / Meals: _______________________________________________

Today's Treatment: ______________________________________________

Today's Small Win: ______________________________________________

## CARE TEAM & NOTES

Nurse(s): __________________ Provider(s): __________________

Questions/Notes:

_______________________________________________________________

_______________________________________________________________

_______________________________________________________________

_______________________________________________________________

_______________________________________________________________

_______________________________________________________________

_______________________________________________________________

# Health Tracker

Date: ________ Day: Su M Tu W Th F Sa

**LABS & VITALS**

WBC: ______ Hemoglobin: ________ Platelets: ________ ANC: __________

Other: _____________ Other: ____________ Other: ______________

Temp: __________ Weight: __________ Other Vitals: ___________________

**SYMPTOMS**

Pain (0-10): ____ Fatigue (0-10): ____ Nausea (0-10): ____

Other (Rash, GI, Mouth Sores, etc.): ________________________________

**DAILY LIVING**

Sleep: ____ hrs Water: ______ oz BM: ______

Movement: ______________________________________________________

Appetite / Meals: ________________________________________________

Today's Treatment: _______________________________________________

Today's Small Win: _______________________________________________

**CARE TEAM & NOTES**

Nurse(s): _________________ Provider(s): _________________

Questions/Notes:

______________________________________________________________

______________________________________________________________

______________________________________________________________

______________________________________________________________

______________________________________________________________

______________________________________________________________

______________________________________________________________

# Health Tracker

Date: ________

Day: Su M Tu W Th F Sa

## LABS & VITALS

WBC: ______ Hemoglobin: ________ Platelets: ________ ANC: __________

Other: ____________ Other: ____________ Other: ______________

Temp: __________ Weight: __________ Other Vitals: ___________________

## SYMPTOMS

Pain (0-10): ____ Fatigue (0-10): ____ Nausea (0-10): ____

Other (Rash, GI, Mouth Sores, etc.): ______________________________

## DAILY LIVING

Sleep: ____ hrs Water: ______ oz BM: ______

Movement: ____________________________________________

Appetite / Meals: ______________________________________

Today's Treatment: _____________________________________

Today's Small Win: _____________________________________

## CARE TEAM & NOTES

Nurse(s): _________________ Provider(s): _________________

Questions/Notes:

______________________________________________________

______________________________________________________

______________________________________________________

______________________________________________________

______________________________________________________

______________________________________________________

______________________________________________________

# Health Tracker

Date: ________ Day: Su M Tu W Th F Sa

## LABS & VITALS

WBC: ______ Hemoglobin: ________ Platelets: ________ ANC: __________

Other: _____________ Other: ____________ Other: ______________

Temp: __________ Weight: __________ Other Vitals: ____________________

## SYMPTOMS

Pain (0-10): ____ Fatigue (0-10): ____ Nausea (0-10): ____

Other (Rash, GI, Mouth Sores, etc.): ________________________________

## DAILY LIVING

Sleep: ____ hrs Water: ______ oz BM: ______

Movement: ______________________________________________________

Appetite / Meals: ________________________________________________

Today's Treatment: _______________________________________________

Today's Small Win: _______________________________________________

## CARE TEAM & NOTES

Nurse(s): _________________ Provider(s): _________________

Questions/Notes:

_______________________________________________________________

_______________________________________________________________

_______________________________________________________________

_______________________________________________________________

_______________________________________________________________

_______________________________________________________________

_______________________________________________________________

# Health Tracker

Date: ________ Day: Su M Tu W Th F Sa

## LABS & VITALS

WBC: ______ Hemoglobin: ________ Platelets: ________ ANC: __________

Other: _____________ Other: ____________ Other: ______________

Temp: __________ Weight: __________ Other Vitals: ___________________

## SYMPTOMS

Pain (0-10): ____ Fatigue (0-10): ____ Nausea (0-10): ____

Other (Rash, GI, Mouth Sores, etc.): ________________________________

## DAILY LIVING

Sleep: ____ hrs Water: ______ oz BM: ______

Movement: ____________________________________________________

Appetite / Meals: ______________________________________________

Today's Treatment: _____________________________________________

Today's Small Win: _____________________________________________

## CARE TEAM & NOTES

Nurse(s): _________________ Provider(s): _________________

Questions/Notes:

____________________________________________________________

____________________________________________________________

____________________________________________________________

____________________________________________________________

____________________________________________________________

____________________________________________________________

____________________________________________________________

# Health Tracker

Date: ________ Day: Su M Tu W Th F Sa

## LABS & VITALS

WBC: ______ Hemoglobin: ________ Platelets: ________ ANC: __________

Other: _____________ Other: ____________ Other: ______________

Temp: __________ Weight: __________ Other Vitals: ___________________

## SYMPTOMS

Pain (0-10): ____ Fatigue (0-10): ____ Nausea (0-10): ____

Other (Rash, GI, Mouth Sores, etc.): ________________________________

## DAILY LIVING

Sleep: ____ hrs Water: ______ oz BM: ______

Movement: ____________________________________________________

Appetite / Meals: ______________________________________________

Today's Treatment: _____________________________________________

Today's Small Win: _____________________________________________

## CARE TEAM & NOTES

Nurse(s): _________________ Provider(s): _________________

Questions/Notes:

______________________________________________________________

______________________________________________________________

______________________________________________________________

______________________________________________________________

______________________________________________________________

______________________________________________________________

______________________________________________________________

# Health Tracker

Date: ________

Day: Su M Tu W Th F Sa

## LABS & VITALS

WBC: ______ Hemoglobin: ________ Platelets: ________ ANC: __________

Other: _____________ Other: ____________ Other: ______________

Temp: __________ Weight: __________ Other Vitals: ___________________

## SYMPTOMS

Pain (0-10): ____ Fatigue (0-10): ____ Nausea (0-10): ____

Other (Rash, GI, Mouth Sores, etc.): ________________________________

## DAILY LIVING

Sleep: ____ hrs Water: ______ oz BM: ______

Movement: ____________________________________________________

Appetite / Meals: ______________________________________________

Today's Treatment: _____________________________________________

Today's Small Win: _____________________________________________

## CARE TEAM & NOTES

Nurse(s): _________________ Provider(s): _________________

Questions/Notes:

_____________________________________________________________

_____________________________________________________________

_____________________________________________________________

_____________________________________________________________

_____________________________________________________________

_____________________________________________________________

_____________________________________________________________

# Health Tracker

Date: ________ Day: Su M Tu W Th F Sa

**LABS & VITALS**

WBC: ______ Hemoglobin: ________ Platelets: ________ ANC: __________

Other: _____________ Other: ____________ Other: ______________

Temp: __________ Weight: __________ Other Vitals: ___________________

**SYMPTOMS**

Pain (0-10): ____ Fatigue (0-10): ____ Nausea (0-10): ____

Other (Rash, GI, Mouth Sores, etc.): _________________________________

**DAILY LIVING**

Sleep: ____ hrs Water: ______ oz BM: ______

Movement: ____________________________________________________

Appetite / Meals: _______________________________________________

Today's Treatment: _____________________________________________

Today's Small Win: _____________________________________________

**CARE TEAM & NOTES**

Nurse(s): _________________ Provider(s): _________________

Questions/Notes:

_______________________________________________________________

_______________________________________________________________

_______________________________________________________________

_______________________________________________________________

_______________________________________________________________

_______________________________________________________________

_______________________________________________________________

# Health Tracker

Date: ________

Day: Su M Tu W Th F Sa

## LABS & VITALS

WBC: ______ Hemoglobin: ________ Platelets: ________ ANC: __________

Other: _____________ Other: ____________ Other: ______________

Temp: __________ Weight: __________ Other Vitals: ___________________

## SYMPTOMS

Pain (0-10): ____ Fatigue (0-10): ____ Nausea (0-10): ____

Other (Rash, GI, Mouth Sores, etc.): ________________________________

## DAILY LIVING

Sleep: ____ hrs Water: ______ oz BM: ______

Movement: ______________________________________________________

Appetite / Meals: ________________________________________________

Today's Treatment: _______________________________________________

Today's Small Win: _______________________________________________

## CARE TEAM & NOTES

Nurse(s): _________________ Provider(s): _________________

Questions/Notes:

_______________________________________________________________

_______________________________________________________________

_______________________________________________________________

_______________________________________________________________

_______________________________________________________________

_______________________________________________________________

_______________________________________________________________

# Health Tracker

Date: ________ Day: Su M Tu W Th F Sa

## LABS & VITALS

WBC: ______ Hemoglobin: ________ Platelets: ________ ANC: __________

Other: _____________ Other: ____________ Other: ______________

Temp: __________ Weight: __________ Other Vitals: ____________________

## SYMPTOMS

Pain (0-10): ____ Fatigue (0-10): ____ Nausea (0-10): ____

Other (Rash, GI, Mouth Sores, etc.): ________________________________

## DAILY LIVING

Sleep: ____ hrs Water: ______ oz BM: ______

Movement: ____________________________________________________

Appetite / Meals: ______________________________________________

Today's Treatment: _____________________________________________

Today's Small Win: _____________________________________________

## CARE TEAM & NOTES

Nurse(s): _________________ Provider(s): _________________

Questions/Notes:

______________________________________________________________

______________________________________________________________

______________________________________________________________

______________________________________________________________

______________________________________________________________

______________________________________________________________

______________________________________________________________

# Health Tracker

Date: ________

Day: Su M Tu W Th F Sa

## LABS & VITALS

WBC: ______ Hemoglobin: ________ Platelets: ________ ANC: __________

Other: _____________ Other: ____________ Other: ______________

Temp: __________ Weight: __________ Other Vitals: ___________________

## SYMPTOMS

Pain (0-10): ____ Fatigue (0-10): ____ Nausea (0-10): ____

Other (Rash, GI, Mouth Sores, etc.): ________________________________

## DAILY LIVING

Sleep: ____ hrs Water: ______ oz BM: ______

Movement: ____________________________________________________

Appetite / Meals: _______________________________________________

Today's Treatment: ______________________________________________

Today's Small Win: ______________________________________________

## CARE TEAM & NOTES

Nurse(s): __________________ Provider(s): _________________

Questions/Notes:

______________________________________________________________

______________________________________________________________

______________________________________________________________

______________________________________________________________

______________________________________________________________

______________________________________________________________

______________________________________________________________

# Health Tracker

Date: ________

Day: Su M Tu W Th F Sa

**LABS & VITALS**

WBC: ______ Hemoglobin: ________ Platelets: ________ ANC: __________

Other: _____________ Other: ____________ Other: ______________

Temp: __________ Weight: __________ Other Vitals: ____________________

**SYMPTOMS**

Pain (0-10): ____ Fatigue (0-10): ____ Nausea (0-10): ____

Other (Rash, GI, Mouth Sores, etc.): __________________________________

**DAILY LIVING**

Sleep: ____ hrs Water: ______ oz BM: ______

Movement: ______________________________________________________

Appetite / Meals: ________________________________________________

Today's Treatment: _______________________________________________

Today's Small Win: _______________________________________________

**CARE TEAM & NOTES**

Nurse(s): _________________ Provider(s): _________________

Questions/Notes:

_______________________________________________________________

_______________________________________________________________

_______________________________________________________________

_______________________________________________________________

_______________________________________________________________

_______________________________________________________________

_______________________________________________________________

# Health Tracker

Date: ________ Day: Su M Tu W Th F Sa

## LABS & VITALS

WBC: ______ Hemoglobin: ________ Platelets: ________ ANC: __________

Other: _____________ Other: ____________ Other: ______________

Temp: __________ Weight: __________ Other Vitals: ___________________

## SYMPTOMS

Pain (0-10): ____ Fatigue (0-10): ____ Nausea (0-10): ____

Other (Rash, GI, Mouth Sores, etc.): ________________________________

## DAILY LIVING

Sleep: ____ hrs Water: ______ oz BM: ______

Movement: ____________________________________________________

Appetite / Meals: ______________________________________________

Today's Treatment: _____________________________________________

Today's Small Win: _____________________________________________

## CARE TEAM & NOTES

Nurse(s): _________________ Provider(s): _________________

Questions/Notes:

_____________________________________________________________

_____________________________________________________________

_____________________________________________________________

_____________________________________________________________

_____________________________________________________________

_____________________________________________________________

_____________________________________________________________

# Health Tracker

Date: ________

Day: Su M Tu W Th F Sa

## LABS & VITALS

WBC: ______ Hemoglobin: ________ Platelets: ________ ANC: __________

Other: _____________ Other: ____________ Other: ______________

Temp: __________ Weight: __________ Other Vitals: ____________________

## SYMPTOMS

Pain (0-10): ____ Fatigue (0-10): ____ Nausea (0-10): ____

Other (Rash, GI, Mouth Sores, etc.): _________________________________

## DAILY LIVING

Sleep: ____ hrs Water: ______ oz BM: ______

Movement: ____________________________________________

Appetite / Meals: ______________________________________

Today's Treatment: _____________________________________

Today's Small Win: _____________________________________

## CARE TEAM & NOTES

Nurse(s): _________________ Provider(s): _________________

Questions/Notes:

_______________________________________________________________

_______________________________________________________________

_______________________________________________________________

_______________________________________________________________

_______________________________________________________________

_______________________________________________________________

_______________________________________________________________

# Health Tracker

Date: ________ Day: Su M Tu W Th F Sa

## LABS & VITALS

WBC: ______ Hemoglobin: ________ Platelets: ________ ANC: __________

Other: _____________ Other: ____________ Other: ______________

Temp: __________ Weight: __________ Other Vitals: ___________________

## SYMPTOMS

Pain (0-10): ____ Fatigue (0-10): ____ Nausea (0-10): ____

Other (Rash, GI, Mouth Sores, etc.): ________________________________

## DAILY LIVING

Sleep: ____ hrs Water: ______ oz BM: ______

Movement: ____________________________________________________

Appetite / Meals: ______________________________________________

Today's Treatment: _____________________________________________

Today's Small Win: _____________________________________________

## CARE TEAM & NOTES

Nurse(s): _________________ Provider(s): _________________

Questions/Notes:

______________________________________________________________

______________________________________________________________

______________________________________________________________

______________________________________________________________

______________________________________________________________

______________________________________________________________

______________________________________________________________

# Health Tracker

Date: ________ Day: Su M Tu W Th F Sa

## LABS & VITALS

WBC: ______ Hemoglobin: ________ Platelets: ________ ANC: __________
Other: _____________ Other: ____________ Other: ______________

Temp: __________ Weight: __________ Other Vitals: ___________________

## SYMPTOMS

Pain (0-10): ____ Fatigue (0-10): ____ Nausea (0-10): ____
Other (Rash, GI, Mouth Sores, etc.): ________________________________

## DAILY LIVING

Sleep: ____ hrs Water: ______ oz BM: ______
Movement: ____________________________________________________
Appetite / Meals: ______________________________________________
Today's Treatment: _____________________________________________
Today's Small Win: _____________________________________________

## CARE TEAM & NOTES

Nurse(s): _________________ Provider(s): _________________
Questions/Notes:

____________________________________________________________
____________________________________________________________
____________________________________________________________
____________________________________________________________
____________________________________________________________
____________________________________________________________
____________________________________________________________

# Health Tracker

Date: ________ Day: Su M Tu W Th F Sa

## LABS & VITALS

WBC: ______ Hemoglobin: ________ Platelets: ________ ANC: __________

Other: _____________ Other: ____________ Other: ______________

Temp: __________ Weight: __________ Other Vitals: ___________________

## SYMPTOMS

Pain (0-10): ____ Fatigue (0-10): ____ Nausea (0-10): ____

Other (Rash, GI, Mouth Sores, etc.): ________________________________

## DAILY LIVING

Sleep: ____ hrs Water: ______ oz BM: ______

Movement: ____________________________________________________

Appetite / Meals: ______________________________________________

Today's Treatment: _____________________________________________

Today's Small Win: _____________________________________________

## CARE TEAM & NOTES

Nurse(s): _________________ Provider(s): _________________

Questions/Notes:

______________________________________________________________

______________________________________________________________

______________________________________________________________

______________________________________________________________

______________________________________________________________

______________________________________________________________

______________________________________________________________

# Health Tracker

Date: ________ Day: Su M Tu W Th F Sa

## LABS & VITALS

WBC: ______ Hemoglobin: ________ Platelets: ________ ANC: __________

Other: _____________ Other: ____________ Other: ______________

Temp: __________ Weight: __________ Other Vitals: ____________________

## SYMPTOMS

Pain (0-10): ____ Fatigue (0-10): ____ Nausea (0-10): ____

Other (Rash, GI, Mouth Sores, etc.): __________________________________

## DAILY LIVING

Sleep: ____ hrs Water: ______ oz BM: ______

Movement: ______________________________________________________

Appetite / Meals: _________________________________________________

Today's Treatment: ________________________________________________

Today's Small Win: ________________________________________________

## CARE TEAM & NOTES

Nurse(s): _________________ Provider(s): _________________

Questions/Notes:

______________________________________________________________

______________________________________________________________

______________________________________________________________

______________________________________________________________

______________________________________________________________

______________________________________________________________

______________________________________________________________

# Health Tracker

Date: ________

Day: Su M Tu W Th F Sa

**LABS & VITALS**

WBC: ______ Hemoglobin: ________ Platelets: ________ ANC: __________

Other: _____________ Other: ____________ Other: ______________

Temp: __________ Weight: __________ Other Vitals: ___________________

**SYMPTOMS**

Pain (0-10): ____ Fatigue (0-10): ____ Nausea (0-10): ____

Other (Rash, GI, Mouth Sores, etc.): ________________________________

**DAILY LIVING**

Sleep: ____ hrs Water: ______ oz BM: ______

Movement: ____________________________________________________

Appetite / Meals: ______________________________________________

Today's Treatment: _____________________________________________

Today's Small Win: _____________________________________________

**CARE TEAM & NOTES**

Nurse(s): _________________ Provider(s): _________________

Questions/Notes:

_____________________________________________________________

_____________________________________________________________

_____________________________________________________________

_____________________________________________________________

_____________________________________________________________

_____________________________________________________________

_____________________________________________________________

# Health Tracker

Date: ________ Day: Su M Tu W Th F Sa

## LABS & VITALS

WBC: ______ Hemoglobin: ________ Platelets: ________ ANC: __________

Other: ______________ Other: ____________ Other: ______________

Temp: __________ Weight: __________ Other Vitals: ____________________

## SYMPTOMS

Pain (0-10): ____ Fatigue (0-10): ____ Nausea (0-10): ____

Other (Rash, GI, Mouth Sores, etc.): ______________________________

## DAILY LIVING

Sleep: ____ hrs Water: ______ oz BM: ______

Movement: ______________________________

Appetite / Meals: ______________________________

Today's Treatment: ______________________________

Today's Small Win: ______________________________

## CARE TEAM & NOTES

Nurse(s): ________________ Provider(s): ________________

Questions/Notes:

______________________________

______________________________

______________________________

______________________________

______________________________

______________________________

______________________________

Week of: ___________ # Weekly Health Log

| Day/ Date | Fluid & Nutrition | Sleep & Movement Hrs/Type | Symptoms & Medication Changes | Bowels Type & Frequency | Vitals Temp, BP, etc. |
|---|---|---|---|---|---|
| MON | | | | | |
| TUES | | | | | |
| WED | | | | | |
| THURS | | | | | |
| FRI | | | | | |
| SAT | | | | | |
| SUN | | | | | |

Week of: ____________

# Weekly Health Log

| Day/ Date | Fluid & Nutrition | Sleep & Movement Hrs/Type | Symptoms & Medication Changes | Bowels Type & Frequency | Vitals Temp, BP, etc. |
|---|---|---|---|---|---|
| MON | | | | | |
| TUES | | | | | |
| WED | | | | | |
| THURS | | | | | |
| FRI | | | | | |
| SAT | | | | | |
| SUN | | | | | |

Week of: ____________ **Weekly Health Log**

| Day/ Date | Fluid & Nutrition | Sleep & Movement Hrs/Type | Symptoms & Medication Changes | Bowels Type & Frequency | Vitals Temp, BP, etc. |
|---|---|---|---|---|---|
| MON | | | | | |
| TUES | | | | | |
| WED | | | | | |
| THURS | | | | | |
| FRI | | | | | |
| SAT | | | | | |
| SUN | | | | | |

Week of: ____________

# Weekly Health Log

| Day/ Date | Fluid & Nutrition | Sleep & Movement Hrs/Type | Symptoms & Medication Changes | Bowels Type & Frequency | Vitals Temp, BP, etc. |
|---|---|---|---|---|---|
| MON | | | | | |
| TUES | | | | | |
| WED | | | | | |
| THURS | | | | | |
| FRI | | | | | |
| SAT | | | | | |
| SUN | | | | | |

Week of: ____________

# Weekly Health Log

| Day/ Date | Fluid & Nutrition | Sleep & Movement Hrs/Type | Symptoms & Medication Changes | Bowels Type & Frequency | Vitals Temp, BP, etc. |
|---|---|---|---|---|---|
| MON | | | | | |
| TUES | | | | | |
| WED | | | | | |
| THURS | | | | | |
| FRI | | | | | |
| SAT | | | | | |
| SUN | | | | | |

Week of: ____________ 

# Weekly Health Log

| Day/ Date | Fluid & Nutrition | Sleep & Movement Hrs/Type | Symptoms & Medication Changes | Bowels Type & Frequency | Vitals Temp, BP, etc. |
|---|---|---|---|---|---|
| MON | | | | | |
| TUES | | | | | |
| WED | | | | | |
| THURS | | | | | |
| FRI | | | | | |
| SAT | | | | | |
| SUN | | | | | |

Week of: ___________

# Weekly Health Log

| Day/ Date | Fluid & Nutrition | Sleep & Movement Hrs/Type | Symptoms & Medication Changes | Bowels Type & Frequency | Vitals Temp, BP, etc. |
|---|---|---|---|---|---|
| MON | | | | | |
| TUES | | | | | |
| WED | | | | | |
| THURS | | | | | |
| FRI | | | | | |
| SAT | | | | | |
| SUN | | | | | |

Week of: ____________

# Weekly Health Log

| Day/ Date | Fluid & Nutrition | Sleep & Movement Hrs/Type | Symptoms & Medication Changes | Bowels Type & Frequency | Vitals Temp, BP, etc. |
|---|---|---|---|---|---|
| MON | | | | | |
| TUES | | | | | |
| WED | | | | | |
| THURS | | | | | |
| FRI | | | | | |
| SAT | | | | | |
| SUN | | | | | |

Week of: ____________

# Weekly Health Log

| Day/ Date | Fluid & Nutrition | Sleep & Movement Hrs/Type | Symptoms & Medication Changes | Bowels Type & Frequency | Vitals Temp, BP, etc. |
|---|---|---|---|---|---|
| MON | | | | | |
| TUES | | | | | |
| WED | | | | | |
| THURS | | | | | |
| FRI | | | | | |
| SAT | | | | | |
| SUN | | | | | |

Week of: ____________ 

# Weekly Health Log

| Day/ Date | Fluid & Nutrition | Sleep & Movement Hrs/Type | Symptoms & Medication Changes | Bowels Type & Frequency | Vitals Temp, BP, etc. |
|---|---|---|---|---|---|
| MON | | | | | |
| TUES | | | | | |
| WED | | | | | |
| THURS | | | | | |
| FRI | | | | | |
| SAT | | | | | |
| SUN | | | | | |

Week of: ____________ 

# Weekly Health Log

| Day/ Date | Fluid & Nutrition | Sleep & Movement Hrs/Type | Symptoms & Medication Changes | Bowels Type & Frequency | Vitals Temp, BP, etc. |
|---|---|---|---|---|---|
| MON | | | | | |
| TUES | | | | | |
| WED | | | | | |
| THURS | | | | | |
| FRI | | | | | |
| SAT | | | | | |
| SUN | | | | | |

Week of: ____________

# Weekly Health Log

| Day/ Date | Fluid & Nutrition | Sleep & Movement Hrs/Type | Symptoms & Medication Changes | Bowels Type & Frequency | Vitals Temp, BP, etc. |
|---|---|---|---|---|---|
| MON | | | | | |
| TUES | | | | | |
| WED | | | | | |
| THURS | | | | | |
| FRI | | | | | |
| SAT | | | | | |
| SUN | | | | | |

# Recommended Reading & References

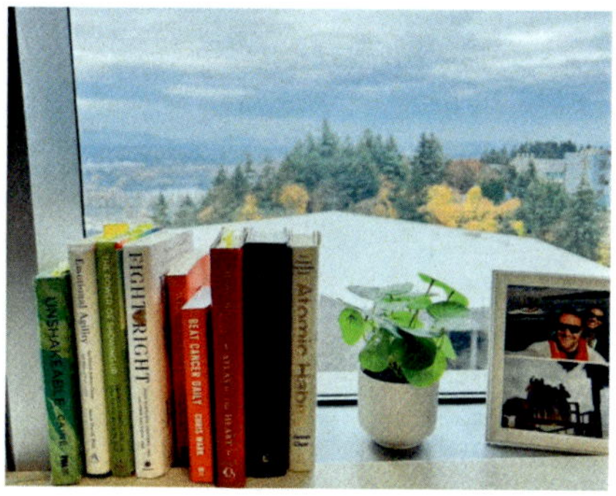

The strategies and tools in this companion are born from our lived experience, but they are also deeply rooted in clinical research, psychology, and neuroscience. If you want to dive deeper into the science of healing, resilience, and connection, here are the experts and resources that guided our journey:

### On Mindset, Grief, and Emotional Resilience:

- Brené Brown: Researcher and author whose work on vulnerability and gratitude profoundly shaped our daily practices.
- David Kessler: World-renowned grief expert and author of Finding Meaning: The Sixth Stage of Grief. His insights on "anticipatory grief" are vital for patients and care partners navigating a diagnosis.
- Kristin Neff: A pioneer in the field of self-compassion. Her work teaches the vital practice of treating yourself with the same grace, kindness, and understanding that you would offer a good friend on your hardest days.
- Lucy Hone: Author of Resilient Grieving. This is an incredibly practical book that focuses on finding strength, adapting to loss, and actively participating in your own healing process.
- Dan Siegel & Tina Payne Bryson: Authors of The Whole-Brain Child. Their frameworks (like "Name it to Tame it" and "Feel Felt") are incredible tools for calming the nervous system during medical trauma.
- Christine Caine: Author of Unshakeable: 365 Devotions for Finding Unwavering Strength. This devotional was a daily anchor. Lindsey read it every single morning to find hope before the hospital day began.

### On Marriage and Connection:

- Dr. John Gottman: Psychological researcher and author of The Seven Principles for Making Marriage Work. His research on the physiological benefits of a "20-Second Hug" helped us stay connected as a couple in the hospital.

### On the Healing Power of Your Environment:

- Dr. Roger Ulrich: A pioneer in Evidence-Based Healthcare Design. His landmark 1984 research in the journal Science proved that a patient's physical environment (like seeing nature, having personal comforts, and reducing clinical noise) directly lowers blood pressure, reduces the perception of pain, and accelerates recovery.

# About the Authors

## Thomas Kealey, RN

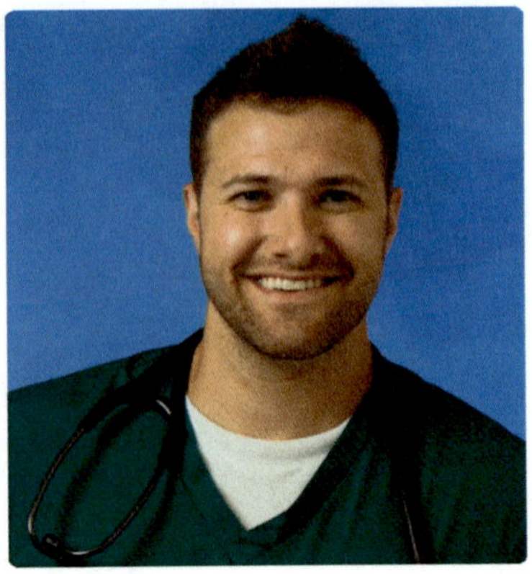

Thomas is a dedicated Registered Nurse and co-host of The Brain it On! Podcast. He combines clinical expertise with deep personal insights from his battle with Multiple Phenotype Acute Leukemia (MPAL). Having navigated a high-risk diagnosis, a stem cell transplant, and a central nervous system relapse, Thomas is passionate about helping patients bridge the gap between clinical care and personal resilience. Currently in remission, he continues to apply the "Brain it On!" strategies to the complexities of post-transplant life.

## Lindsey Kealey, MAT

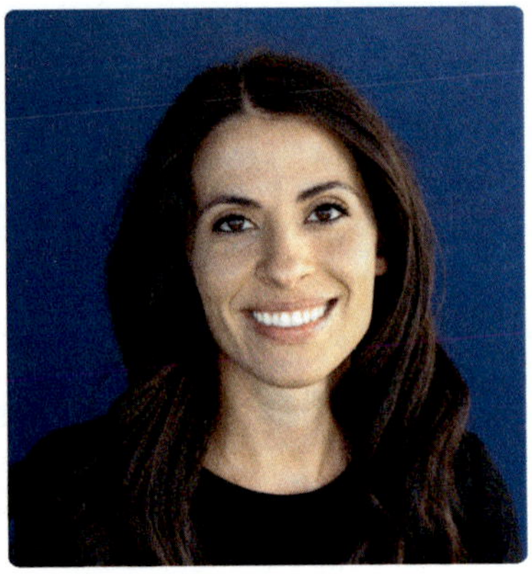

Lindsey is an instructor of Human Development and Family Sciences at Oregon State University and the author of PAWsitive Choices Social and Emotional Learning. With a background in elementary and higher education, she developed a curriculum that integrates neuroscience and problem-solving to foster resilience in children and families. As the co-host of The Brain it On! Podcast, she translates her professional expertise into practical strategies for caregivers, helping them navigate the emotional and logistical adversity of a medical crisis.

## The Journey Behind the Book

The Comfort & Healing Companion was born in a hospital room at Oregon Health & Science University. In 2024, the Kealey family was hit with back-to-back challenges: Thomas' mother, Julie, was diagnosed with late-stage pancreatic cancer, followed just three months later by Thomas' own leukemia diagnosis on Lindsey and Thomas' 10th anniversary.

Witnessing the mutual support between a mother and son fighting cancer simultaneously inspired The Brain it On! Podcast. This toolkit is a collection of the resources they relied on and the strategies they developed to find control, comfort, and even joy amidst the most difficult clinical environments.

# Digital Resource Library

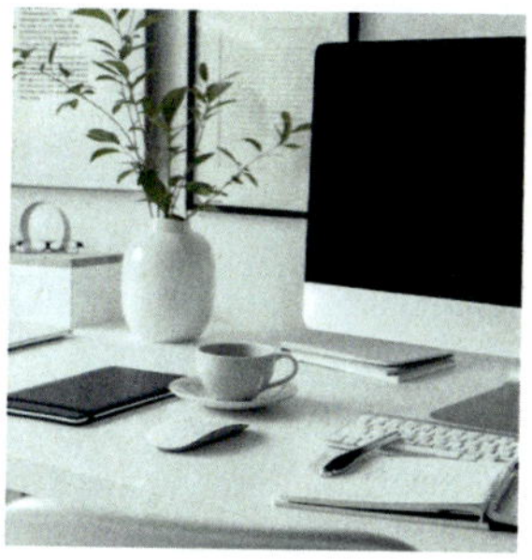

To support your ongoing recovery, we have created an exclusive digital library for our readers featuring:

- **Companion Video Tutorials** to walk you through the strategies
- **Printable Trackers** for health, gratitude, small wins, and care team connections
- **Recommended Support Items** with hyperlinks that take you to our favorites
- **Kids' Resources** to support their emotional needs
- **Faith-Based Encouragement** that anchored our family during treatment
- **Podcast Episodes** that support ideas in the book

To access these resources, scan the QR code or visit:
www.comfortandhealing.org/resources

We truly hope this guide brings you comfort, practical help, and a renewed sense of hope on your health journey. Remember, you're not alone, and every step, no matter how small, is a victory worth celebrating. Be sure to connect with us and become part of our community! You can find more resources, encouragement, and new episodes on our various platforms.

**If this book has helped you, please scan the QR code above or visit our website to leave a review and share this companion with a friend.**

**Connect With Us:**

- Email: brainitonpodcast@gmail.com
- Instagram: instagram.com/thebrainitonpodcast
- YouTube: youtube.com/@thebrainitonpodcast
- Apple Podcasts and Spotify

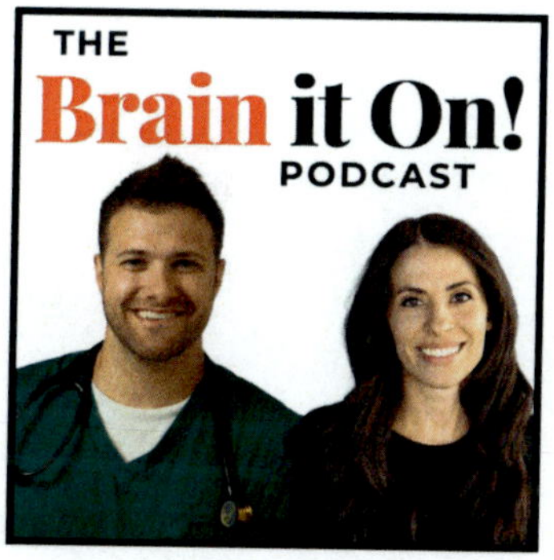


**We're cheering you on!**

*Thomas & Lindsey Kealey*

Made in United States
Orlando, FL
06 November 2026

90240676R00081